COMMITMENT TO HEALTH

My road to recovery and self-discovery fighting chronic pain

JERRY OLYNYK, CLU

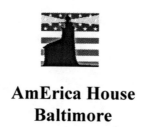

AmErica House
Baltimore

First printing

ISBN: 1-58851-682-2
PUBLISHED BY AMERICA HOUSE BOOK PUBLISHERS
www.publishamerica.com
Baltimore

Printed in the United States of America

To my wife Sasha I dedicate this book
Who in love
Was challenged
With forces unknown
She won the battle for the story to be told

Acknowledgments

To Eileen Molnar who has seen the project from its beginnings. Typing and transposing my handwritten notes which were written under difficult conditions was a feat in itself.

To Brian Scrivener who read and critiqued the original work. For me as a first time writer of a book, initially it was difficult to comprehend why it needed tightening up as I felt everything I had written was important. I quickly realized that Brian was concerned about what the reader wants. His suggestions were most valuable and appreciated.

To Audrey McClellan who took the job of doing the substantive edit and preparing it into its final form. Her probing mind had many questions to be answered and/or clarified from the original text. With a lot of communication, she persevered, tightened it up and brought it to completion.

Terri Elderton who did the copy edit made some timely and valuable contributions to the make up of the final text.

To Dr. Marlene Hunter, Dr. Robert Keyes, Dr. Stuart McNeil and Dr. May Ong for taking the time to review the work and for your endorsements. A special thanks to Dr. Marlene Hunter and Dr. Stuart McNeil for your guidance in some highly technical areas. Also for Dr McNeil's contribution of an illustration showing Anterior Cervical Fusions. To Dr. Ron Bull who has been my personal physician since moving to Chilliwack, his testimonial is reflected in the type of care and guidance which he provided me through some very troubled times.

To Nazlan Khamis who has been my pharmacist since our move in 1991 to Chilliwack. I am grateful for having her as a pharmacist and her guidance during some very troubled times. Her willingness to review the manuscript and do an endorsement is a tribute as it is to all others.

To my colleagues, Moe Bardos, Alan Clapp and Jim Rogers, who all knew me prior to my health problem. To Moe Bardos and Alan Clapp a special thanks for your input.

To Dr. Shirley Baker Thomas, Dr. Clive Duncan, Dr. J. McFadden, Dr. Mike Sookochoff and Linda Thorson for taking the time to do a review.

To our son, John, whose place of work was distant from our home during my critical illness for the first time learned what his parents had gone through.

To everyone my gracious thanks for your testimonials. I did not know what to expect when my written word was to be reviewed by such a fine group of people, however, your support has made me feel like my efforts were worthwhile.

Last but not least a special love and thank you to my wife, Sasha, to whom I dedicate this book.

The demands on her as a caregiver will never fully be known, she saw me happy, she saw me sad, she saw me in pain like I never had, she persevered as did I, a wedding vow is more than meets the eye.

TESTIMONIALS

I have had the opportunity to review this manuscript. I also had the opportunity to evaluate this patient at the height of his medical difficulties. The patient's account of his difficulties and his abilities to overcome those disabilities is a testament to the determination of the patient himself. This journal reflects the nature of this patient's journey for illness to health. This journal also emphasizes how important a positive attitude can be in determining the final outcome from any medical condition.

I also had the opportunity to meet with this patient several years after his illness. It was amazing to see the difference in this patient over that time period. The patient's physical health clearly reflects the changes that have occurred in this patient over the years he has journeyed from illness back to health.

I recommend this book to all individuals who are coping with long-standing pain syndromes of any time.

Robert D. Keyes, M.D., F.R.C.P.(C)

* * *

Rarely does one have the opportunity to travel along a journey of chronic pain, with the one who has been there. *Commitment to Health - My Road to Recovery and Self Discovery Fighting Chronic Pain* offers the reader this unique privilege. In a saga which spans many years, we find ourselves caught up in the day-to-day small joys and mighty miseries of such a journey – and we come to realize that the small joys are what keep us human. It is a testament to courage and determination.

We also are offered an important lifestyle message: to survive, to overcome, to live, keep walking. We would all do well to remember it.

Dr. Marlene Hunter, M.D., F.C.F.P.(C)

* * *

Jerry Olynyk's story deserves to be heard by anyone who has experienced a significant injury due to a motor vehicle accident.

We recognize that the vast majority of these injuries will resolve within a relatively short period of time – treated or untreated.

A small percentage of injured persons will have lingering problems, but tolerable and non-disabling.

A very few injured persons will have long term disability problems – Mr. Olynyk clearly developed long term problems after his motor vehicle accident. Despite his severe symptoms he did try to continue working. Eventually, after considerable time and almost all forms of conservative therapy, surgery was recommended. This was a very difficult decision. Were the symptom and disability genuine? Would surgery be the answer to cure the significant problem and eliminate the disability? No one knew for certain the answer to the questions. But, in the final analysis it is a decision that has to be made by the patient and the surgeon. As I told Mr. Olynyk, "the proof is in the pudding."

His narrative describes very well and in great detail the problems that confront injured persons, lawyers, physicians and insurance companies especially in the framework of a litigious society.

Dr. Stuart McNeil, M.D., B.A., F.R.C.S. (C)

* * *

I would like to congratulate you on completing your book telling of your recovery and self-discovery while fighting chronic pain for well over a decade.

Your book about how you survived under constant excruciating pain should be inspirational reading for anyone. I should know; your struggle was in itself an inspiration; and, I was witness to it all.

I am glad to see you finish your manuscript. The book will be of special help to someone who is now in severe pain and feels so alone.

M.A. Bardos
Life Insurance Broker (& Lawyer - Member of the BC Bar)

* * *

A compelling story. You have shown an inordinate amount of courage and patience. Continued better health.

James E. Rogers, B.A., MBA, CFP, RFP, CHFC
The Rogers Group - Financial Advisors

* * *

It has been a true privilege to be allowed to review this manuscript. Your tenacious persistence and sometimes insurmountable hurdles in your fight to recover from immense pain and devastation in lifestyle have been truly remarkable. You took what fate handed to you, put faith in the medical community, and made a commitment to fitness. Recovery is not easy, as you well found out, and one is never truly recovered, but you and Sasha have both managed to grow from this. As I turned each page, I could feel your pain and suffering. I marveled at your understanding of the medical aspects of your condition. You are a true inspiration for all those people suffering every day, and lost in the bureaucracy of our medical system. I pray they too will be inspired.

Nazlin Khamis, B. Sc. Pharm.
Pharmacy Proprietor

* * *

Commitment to Health is a compelling story of an individual's struggle with the lifestyle changes that follow a significant injury. It is a very personal journey of many years through chronic pain, through our medical system, and through the inevitable paperwork that confronts a person in such a situation.

Jerry Olynyk has been able to get through all of this by the wonderful approach that he has developed to meet these challenges. He presents a story of active involvement, determination, intelligent questioning and research and, most of all, resistance to being swallowed up by an affliction. His work will be an inspiration to any individuals and families who are dealing with long-term problems.

Commitment to Health also offers much to those who enjoy full health. Jerry Olynyk's approach to healthful living can benefit anyone.

One also cannot overlook the tremendous benefit of a supportive spouse and family. I congratulate Jerry and his wife Sasha.

Ronald K. Bull, M.Sc., M.D.

* * *

Jerry Olynyk's *Commitment to Health* provides many new insights to handling pain and continued good health. I am inspired and impressed with his insight and perseverance. It should be read by everyone in the health care system, especially pain clinic professionals as well as those who are providers and marketer's of disability insurance.

Allen Clapp,
Financial and Retirement
Planning Consultant

* * *

Dear Mr. Olynyk,

"His story exemplifies one's determination to rise above his pain and to gain control of life once again in spite of the pain."

Yours truly,
Dr. May Ong, B.Sc., M.D., F.R.C.P.(C)

* * *

The book tells the story and is something I could never have imagined that my mom and dad had gone through. I love you both so much and admire your love for one another. You have taken love to another level. I see so many people who are injured, and with disabilities, and the wife or husband leaves due to coping problems. Not unlike yourselves, I have workers whose spouses have stayed with them, the reason why – "for the love of this person", is what they all tell me.

You are both amazing.

Love,
John

COMMITMENT TO HEALTH

CONTENTS

Introduction

COMMITMENT TO HEALTH

I began writing this book in the early 1980s. I had started a program of healthy eating and exercise and wanted to share my experience with others if my self-imposed program was successful.

In the 1980s, North America was becoming a health-conscious society, but this consciousness was not for everyone. Many of us were too busy with our own lives and all too often we did not worry about our health until something drastic happened to us or, if we were lucky, we awakened in time to smell the coffee burning.

I was in the second category. My wife Sasha and I had married in the early 1950s and enjoyed a happy, stable marriage with six children. I was an executive in an insurance office, doing a lot of entertaining, working long days but finding it fulfilling.

As is often the case when one enjoys the good life with no real worries except taking care of daily challenges, I slowly but surely put a lot of excess weight on my five-foot, six-inch frame. Over a period of twenty-two years I had gone gradually from a slim, trim 160 pounds to a weight of 210 and gaining. Whenever I was being measured by my tailor for a new suit, he would be adding a little cloth, fractions here and there, but never making an issue of it except perhaps for a joke about the fact that I had gained a little weight. My response to the tailor was always, "Do not make it too loose because I am going to lose some weight."

I kept telling my tailor I was going to lose some weight, but on reflection it seems strange that I was not discussing this with my personal physician. After all, who can best put you on track: your doctor or your tailor?

My lifestyle was similar to that of many: I had a good home life, worked full throttle, put in long days, and led a sedentary lifestyle. Had my body had as much exercise as my brain, I am positive that I would not have been carrying all of that excess weight. Ironically, I was in the life insurance business, a business that is directly related to health and risk factors, so I was talking and thinking about these issues every day. But I was not applying them to myself.

This is not to say that my wife and I, as well as our family together, did not enjoy a game of tennis, a game of golf, cross-country skiing, going for a walk, cycling, ice skating, and bowling. In addition, over the years I had coached box lacrosse and ice hockey. Yes, I was active, or so I thought. However, there is a difference between casual activities and a disciplined daily exercise routine.

Although I had long been aware of the fact that our bodies require daily exercise, I had ignored this critical daily regime. I did not have a daily physical fitness program, nor did I follow a program of healthy eating. We ate our three meals a day – in my case probably three plus, what with the snacking habit – but were we eating the right foods? I didn't know or understand the concept of "This food is good for me; this food is not good for me" and didn't worry at all about putting bad food into the engine that kept me running. I had grown fat and sassy eating too many of the wrong foods and not using enough physical energy to burn them off. Without a doubt, you need the combination of good foods as well as the physical exercise to keep you fit.

In early summer 1984, Sasha and I were preparing to leave for a company convention when, as a matter of routine, I arranged for a medical checkup with my personal physician. It was a last-minute item, late Friday afternoon, and we were leaving the following morning.

After the doctor took a third blood pressure reading and appeared to be greatly concerned, I asked him if there was something wrong with his blood pressure monitor. He assured me it was in perfect working order but that my blood pressure reading was very high – 200 over 110 – that my weight was 210 pounds, and that in his opinion I was not in shape to pass an insurance medical. What a bombshell the day before a major trip.

We discussed the situation and I asked if we should cancel our trip. The doctor said no. He would put me on some medication that would keep things under control until we came back, but he cautioned me about getting caught in a situation where I might overexert myself, where I might have cause to grab my luggage and run with it to catch a plane – where too much excitement might cause a heart attack!

He further cautioned me to take it easy but enjoy the trip and not live in fear. This was certainly not the best way to prepare to leave on a trip, but as long as it had the doctor's blessing that was good enough for me.

The doctor's comment that I would not pass an insurance medical really got to me, especially since I worked in insurance. I knew a company would insure me, but not at a standard rate. I could get a policy, but would have to pay a higher premium due to the additional risk factor of high blood pressure and overweight. This did not sit well with me.

It is incredible how when you are under pressure, your mind responds. In those critical moments in the doctor's office, the name of Dr. Ken Cooper flashed into my mind. Ken Cooper believes in the "aerobics" of walking and I had heard him as a guest speaker at one of our conventions. At the time I listened to him, I visualized myself as one of the individuals he was speaking to as even then I knew what he had to say was the right thing for me. But it is so easy to listen, much harder to put into practice as we think, "I'm too busy. I don't have the time." Besides, Dr. Cooper's advice seemed too simple – just a few minutes of walking each day – and it certainly threw me off course. I talked myself out of it: "How can walking possibly keep me in shape and provide me with the necessary physical fitness?" Procrastination plus a thousand excuses meant the walking program was never put in place. But right there and then, as I sat in the doctor's office, I made a commitment to initiate a walking program to regain my physical fitness.

I asked my doctor to recommend a book on balanced diets. He suggested *Eat to Win* by Dr. Robert Haas, and I purchased a copy at the airport the next morning prior to our departure. As we settled in for our long flight, Vancouver, B.C., to Paris, France, I was reading the book before takeoff and it occupied me until we got to Paris. By the time we landed I had recognized my poor eating habits, but I was also feeling good because I could already envision myself with a proper diet, walking the pounds away. This idea of walking myself to good health was firmly imprinted on my mind and I made a further commitment: from now on I was going to live a twenty-three-hour day. The twenty-fourth hour, wherever it may be, would be used for aerobic walking.

We had a great convention in Monte Carlo and then set out touring Europe on a three-week Eurail Pass. The travel by rail was restful, and when our destination was quite distant we travelled by night, always arriving in the early hours of the morning in a new city. As we travelled, both my wife and I were conscious of my health condition and took it easy, a careful day at a time.

On our return from vacation I initiated my "Commitment to Health" program. I started taking a daily walk and I started slowly. I had read of many types of exercise programs that went in fits and starts, always ending in collapse. I had read about crash diets. I decided early on that I would not only make a serious commitment but that it would be a long-term one. As long as I was making progress on a monthly basis I would be happy and wouldn't expect immediate change. My commitment to diet and exercise was going to be slow and steady so that once I lost a pound it would stay off.

When I started my daily walks I soon found out that the distance I could walk was limited compared to my expectations. I could not walk very fast and in no time at all I would be wringing with perspiration. Additionally, we lived on a mountainside so the streets were hilly. Just try walking uphill when you are out of shape.

My peak weight was 215 pounds. At that point my suits were big, yet because they were tailor fitted they hid the blubber. My goal was to get back to 160 pounds. It was hard to comprehend that I was on a mission to lose fifty-five pounds. I tried to think of a way to picture the loss of this much weight. Finally I put the fifty-five pounds in perspective. On a grocery shopping trip I stopped at the shelves where sugar was displayed. I counted eleven five-pound bags of sugar, noted the volume, and in total disbelief said to myself, "All of that volume is on my body and I am carrying it around. Little wonder I am perspiring after walking a few blocks."

I decided I would visualize five-pound bags of sugar as the goal increments that I would set out to lose. Five pounds at a time was achievable, fifty-five pounds was downright scary.

Within a few months I knew that my Commitment to Health was working. My walks were extended from fifteen minutes a day to half an hour, to forty-five minutes, and then to an hour four times a week. I was walking a mile in twelve to fifteen minutes, meeting Dr.

Cooper's definition of "aerobic" walking, and I was losing a pound to a pound and a half a month, so I knew that this part of the equation was working. I was elated when I lost my first five pounds and went to the kitchen cupboard to lift the five-pound bag of sugar that I had bought to be my measure of weight loss. Five pounds of sugar may not sound like much, but it is a lot when you are relating it to the weight on your body. One down and ten to go. Easily said, but at the time it suddenly seemed insurmountable. However, foremost in my mind was my Commitment to Health.

The other part of the equation was that Sasha also read the book *Eat to Win* and she implemented the dietary recommendations in the book. I not only had my aerobic walking program underway, but I was also eating properly. It is so important that we don't just eat but that we make absolutely certain that we are taking in the right type of foods in adequate daily amounts.

I was well on my way: I was losing weight, my blood pressure was coming down, and I was feeling great that a disciplined commitment to better health was working.

It took me five years to lose the fifty-five pounds. Of course there were days when I wondered whether or not it would work, but I kept reducing that pile of five-pound bags of sugar until I was 160 pounds. Imagine a pile of eleven five-pound bags of sugar reduced to zero. Walk into any grocery store; if you are carrying excess weight, do as I did and see how many excess five-pound bags of sugar you are carrying. Even if it is a bag or two, it is a lot. When I was down to five, four, three, two, and one to go it was still scary, but it was no longer eleven.

Though I visualized my excess weight as bags of sugar, it is not sugar that must come off but water. There is an old saying: "If you take it off fast, it will come back; take it off slowly and it will stay off." I firmly believe this saying, and it means if we want to lose weight we must deal with long-term, habit-forming discipline.

My Commitment to Health program is now in its seventeenth year. For the past twelve years I have taken my walks seven days a week, an hour and a half each day, rain or shine. (I emphasize rain or shine as it is so easy to talk yourself out of a walk when it is raining. But believe it or not, there are umbrellas so big that you can go for your walk and come home dry – and it is very refreshing.)

We live in the country and there is nothing on earth so beautiful as to hear the birds chirping in the morning, see squirrels crossing the road, eagles soaring overhead, a deer in the pasture, and a red fox chasing a rabbit, and feel the breath of spring as pussy willows break out in bloom. I witnessed the changing seasons with my friend Duchess, a beautiful long-haired German Shepherd, at my side. In 1996 I lost this good friend to arthritis of the hip. Now I walk with Duke, a Belgian Shepherd and a German Shepherd named 'Whoppee' we acquired while Duchess was still alive. They are great companions to each other and also to me.

There is no doubt that I am addicted to my daily aerobic walking. On occasions when my walking was interrupted due to other health problems, it gave me an empty feeling. At this stage, after years of walking, I can say unequivocally that aerobic walking is the best, most accessible exercise and should not be underestimated. I have never read a negative about walking. My experience through some difficult periods with my health was that to get out and walk, not trying to break records, did wonders for me and it will for you.

Walking - and eating - your way to better health

As a result of my Commitment to Health program – which involved both walking and becoming much more aware of the food I ate and how my metabolism functioned – I have benefited beyond words. It was not just the walking and it was not just the eating habits that brought me down from 215 pounds to 160. It was a combination of both and I cannot stress enough how this combination requires a balance. The balance is to nourish your body only to the extent that it requires and with the proper foods. Moreover, it is important to understand how your metabolism works and how your body properly uses the nourishment you give it. Do not lose sight of the fact that you possess a natural system so intricate that we are not able to duplicate it artificially. Do not take your body for granted as I did, feeding it far beyond its needs, improperly at that. I could not handle it and the pounds went on.

I believe one of the finest parts of our anatomy is our taste buds. They tell us when something is sweet or sour or hot and spicy. However, they do not tell us whether something is good for us or not. They take what is given, no questions asked. This is where the junk food manufacturers come in. Their products are not prepared for the food value but for our taste buds, and taste buds being what they are, we will actually salivate at the thought of the junk food. Taste buds have an uncanny way of controlling what we consume. Too often our body acts as a garbage pail for the junk food.

We hear of the high cost of living, but studies have shown that the cost of living can be greatly reduced by having less junk food in the shopping cart. Spend that money on proper nutrition and you will not only save on your shopping costs but will also enjoy a better, healthier quality of life. Replace the junk food with wholesome fresh fruit and put the taste buds to work. You will develop a craving for fresh fruit, which is vital for a healthy, properly functioning constitution.

Anyone who feels that they should do something about eating to keep fit would be well advised to take the initiative and start a self-learning program or enlist the help of a nutritionist. Perhaps your doctor can refer you to a nutritionist who will guide you on the path to better eating habits.

Most health food store proprietors are quite knowledgeable and will lend a hand to help an inquiring mind. They generally display an array of books that may be helpful in getting you started on better eating habits or other areas concerning health. Health food stores are also a source of good food and other items that will help you as you move to a healthier lifestyle.

I highly recommend spending time in any general bookstore, health food store, or library that has a section of books on nutrition and other areas of health you may be interested in. Many of these books are written by doctors or nutritionists, people who have spent many years coming to understand the needs of the human body in terms of nutrition.

As I was in a vocation that involves a degree of socializing, all too often I would eat in a restaurant, ordering what sounded good rather than what was good for me. This is not to say that there was not nutritious food to choose from on a menu at a good establishment, but

I know that the saliva would flow when I read the description of a tasty-sounding entree that I did not need. I would top it off with a great-tasting dessert and then would feel stuffed, overloaded with calories that I would not burn off.

We can indulge in the proper foods in a social situation, but we also need the regimen of an exercise program to keep the body properly nourished. I firmly believe that the best non-prescription drug to enhance digestion is aerobic walking, along with any other disciplined exercise program you may embark on. I know how I feel after a good walk: refreshed, invigorated, and ready to get on with whatever it is I am doing. On the other hand, I know how I feel after leaving the dinner table if I have overeaten. Certainly not refreshed, invigorated, and ready to go except if it's absolutely necessary. All too often we allow ourselves to sit down where it is more comfortable and relax.

All of us, whatever our situation, must ask ourselves what we can do to help ourselves on the road to health. It is a deep commitment and can be selfish, but it will work no matter who you are if you are committed. I have read many articles describing the many ways to stay fit and I have no argument with any of them, albeit some can put certain stresses on the body. (Even walking can be stressful when you start out, and you must be careful not to expect miracles overnight.) Hardly a day goes by when we do not see an article pertaining to health, whatever the specific subject may be, in our daily newspaper. (Ironically, often we read a news item one day that says such-and-such a food item is good for you while the next day we find that it is not.) There are magazines to subscribe to, government publications providing valuable information on health, health food stores, and fitness centers everywhere. There is also your personal physician, who would be more than pleased to give you direction if you wanted to start scheduling a twenty-three-hour day, with the twenty-fourth hour dedicated to walking. These articles and facilities inform us about the foods that are good for us or not good for us, the acceptable levels for proper nutrition and nourishment, the importance of keeping our bodies in condition through some form of physical fitness program.

Unfortunately, all of this information, all these support systems reach only a small percentage of the public. They don't affect those people who because of their lifestyle or for whatever reason do not set aside the time to take stock and do a health inventory occasionally. We get so caught up in our individual lives that sometimes the most important element, our body, is taken for granted and totally neglected. Then suddenly we find out on our own or from our doctor that something is out of balance in our blood; we are tiring beyond the norm or we cannot go the full eighteen holes of golf at the pace we used to. Anyone reading this book who has or has had a health problem will easily relate to what I am saying. All too often a heart attack or stroke could have been avoided if only we knew what was happening on the inside. In many cases there are advance warning signs but we are too busy to heed them. If this book helps only one person in this category, it will have been worth the effort. However, I hope and believe it will help many.

We live in a social climate that offers the best of everything. The best of foods and the tastiest of junk foods – if indeed there is such a thing (we must admit our taste buds tell us so). We live in a society where we all too often eat by impulse, temptation, and taste rather than by determining how much this body can take without being overcharged. We don't ask ourselves, "Will there be the necessary energy expended today to get rid of these unneeded calories?"

We must remember we are not in the Olympics; we are not competing with others for recognition or awards. We are competing with an unhealthy approach to living and must not expect dramatic change in a short amount of time. It takes a long-term commitment to really make a change. When I set my goal of losing fifty-five pounds I may have been unrealistic, not realizing how much commitment this goal would require. However, I set myself a long-term goal and stuck to it. From what I have learned and read over the years, I believe it is the most successful way to achieve good health.

COMMITMENT TO HEALTH

Chapter 1

FIGHT OR FLIGHT

Little did I know that in spite of my commitment to health, in a split second my situation was to change in a way that would ultimately reshape my life for years to come.

In November 1984, on my way to work early in the morning, I was involved in a motor vehicle accident in which I was rear-ended by two cars.

I was wearing a seat belt and for a few moments was in a total daze, knocked out by the impact of the accident. When I got out of my vehicle, the other two drivers were well into a discussion of what had happened and were surveying the damage to the vehicles.

As the accident occurred during rush hour at the ramp onto Lions Gate Bridge, which spans the narrows of Burrard Inlet leading into Vancouver, the three of us agreed that we should drive on to the other side and meet to exchange information at a predetermined location. When I finally got to the office after this I was still dazed, shaking from the trauma of the accident and in pain. I phoned home, told Sasha about the crash, and set about to do my work.

As the day progressed I found my pain increasing and came to the conclusion that there was something seriously wrong with me. I had never felt such pain before. It was centred in my neck, shooting up to my skull, but I also felt pain throughout my body from the shaking and the physical trauma of the accident. I was frightened and overwhelmed by this pain and by my lack of ability to control it.

By the end of my workday I could not help wondering what I was still doing at the office. I don't know how I managed to stay functioning so long. On the way home I dropped in at our medical clinic, hoping that my personal physician was in. He was, and after waiting for him to get through his scheduled appointments (which seemed to take forever), I finally saw him.

Dr. B commented that I'd obviously had a bad jolt. He diagnosed whiplash, gave me some medication, scheduled X-rays, and booked me for a round of physiotherapy, but he concluded that the best healer was time and I'd have to give my neck and body time to settle down.

The drug he prescribed this day was of little help, as were the multitude of other medications prescribed in the months to come. Physiotherapy was actually regressive. I was subjected to many types of treatment at a physiotherapy clinic, all to no avail. Instead they produced increased pain and by the end of December my visits to physio were discontinued.

When Dr. B saw the X-rays, he immediately booked me an appointment with an orthopaedic surgeon. The X-rays showed I had pre-existing disc degeneration and the jolting of the accident had caused acute symptoms. I believe Dr. B wanted an orthopaedic specialist to examine the X-rays and see me due to the more serious nature of the injury and the pain I was enduring.

At the same time this was going on, I also had to deal with an insurance claim. I contacted an insurance adjuster to do an estimate of damage to my car. In his requisition for repairs, the major item that needed to be replaced was my rear bumper. However, there's a big difference between a visual observation, which is what the adjuster did, and a thorough inspection for possible damage. The repair shop did the latter and one of the mechanics called to tell me that the car's frame had been bent from the impact and that he needed to contact the adjuster to get clearance to straighten out the frame.

My car, a new Chrysler New Yorker Fifth Avenue, was big and solid. Consider what must happen to your body, particularly your neck and head, when it is subjected to the force and thrust of an accident that can bend the frame of such a car. The consequences to your body are referred to as whiplash. Generally speaking, whiplash causes soft tissue damage that will heal and settle down on its own over time. In my case, the pre-existing disc condition had been aggravated and was not settling down and any conservative treatment – such as physiotherapy – was only making it worse.

I continued going to work, but I did not have any letup from the skull pain and on January 4, 1985, I saw the orthopaedic surgeon, Dr. Stuart McNeill, for the first time. Dr. McNeill took more X-rays and fitted me with a soft cervical collar. This provided some support for my head and neck, but it was not enough as the pain continued to radiate

26

through the area of my neck to the skull. I was ingesting a steady diet of anti-inflammatory drugs, but they were of little help and I was in a lot of distress.

In a later medical legal report that Dr. McNeill wrote for my insurance claim he stated: "These x-rays [taken on the day of my accident, November 24, 1984] did demonstrate quite severe degenerative changes at the C.4/5 level. There was also some associated changes at the C.6/7 level and perhaps some very minimal changes at C.5/6 but these really were rather insignificant. Indeed on the basis of the plain x-rays, the major problems appeared to be at both the 4/5 and the 6/7 levels.

"At that time it was clear that Mr. Olynyk did in fact have evidence of cervical spondylosis. It was quite obvious that these changes on the x-rays had existed before the motor vehicle accident. My diagnosis at that time was a problem of pre-existing cervical spondylosis which had been asymptomatic and now rendered symptomatic as a result of the motor vehicle accident which occurred on the 8th November 1984. We do recognize that these type of injuries are essentially flexion extension type injuries involving the cervical spine. In some cases the damage appears to be soft tissue in nature, but when a patient does have pre-existing cervical spondylosis, then of course it is well recognized that these previously asymptomatic discs can be rendered symptomatic and this can then result in a symptom complex of neck pain, headaches, stiffness, spasm, as well as other symptoms."

Dr. McNeill said that he was waiting to see if my injuries would settle on their own. Unfortunately, it was not to be. I suffered constant pain for the next two years. I could not control it with the variety of painkillers I was prescribed nor with the soft neck collar I wore.

I continued to work full days though I was getting less accomplished and was not working to my usual standards. From the time I entered the life insurance business in 1962 I had kept a daily diary where I noted appointments as well as detailed records of meetings. Looking back at my daily diary for 1985 and 1986 I see that I was scheduling fewer business appointments and more doctor appointments, and I would sometimes have to leave the office an hour or two early because the pain was so severe. Around this time I started keeping a separate journal where I recorded events related to my insurance claim. As I came to realize that something was seriously wrong with me, this became an accident journal in which I tracked my health condition.

To make matters worse, on July 25, 1985, I was involved in another fender bender on my way home from work. Although it was a very minor accident, it did contribute stress and trauma, adding to the distress I was in from the original collision.

At the request of the Insurance Corporation of BC, which was handling my accident claim, I went to see another orthopaedic surgeon in December 1985. This man wrote in his report on my case: "I do not think this man is going to be helped by surgical treatment either now or in the future. I suggest that he has quite widespread degenerative changes in his cervical spine and operating on one or more levels is unlikely to relieve his symptoms...I think, therefore, that this man has been involved in a relatively minor motor vehicle accident in which he has the familiar symptoms related to this type of injury. I would think that this man's symptoms will improve with his exercise program. He may be one of those people who is left with some residual symptoms related to his neck, but I have found over a period of time that these symptoms do not tend to significantly interfere with the working or recreational activities of the subject. He may therefore have symptoms which I would describe as being of a nuisance value but I do not think he will have a significant disability as a result of this accident."

This doctor also suggested that it would be advisable for me to see a chiropractor. I discussed this with Dr. McNeill and he was disgusted. He said that given the nature of my condition, chiropractic manipulation could cause further complications instead of helping.

In early 1987, Dr. McNeill decided it was time to do a myelogram. In this procedure dye is injected into the spine to highlight the affected area on an X-ray. (In my case it would show if nerves were being pinched.) In the event that surgery is necessary, a myelogram gives the surgeon information so there are no surprises once the operation is underway. This is a more invasive procedure than medication, physiotherapy, and time, but Dr. McNeill felt it was necessary at this stage so he could see what was happening.

I was admitted to Lions Gate Hospital on April 10, 1987, for the myelogram. A radiologist injected dye into my spine and took X-rays of the area. They showed that there was a nerve being pinched at the C4/5 level. The disc between the fourth and fifth vertebrae in my cervical spine was narrowing and it was herniating on the right side. The protrusion from the herniated disc was affecting the nerve (see "A Brief Introduction to the Spine" following this chapter).

Vertebral Column

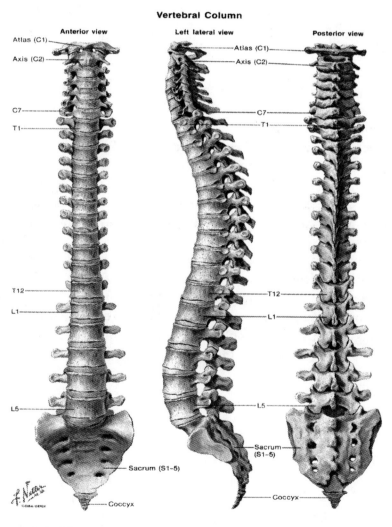

I have included a diagram of the vertebral column because it is the subject matter of this book. I don't intend to identify all the parts of what we know as the backbone or spine. The vertebrae, nerves, spinal cord, discs, facet joints, ligaments, and muscles associated with this structure are complex. It only accounts for about 14 percent of our body weight, but all too often it is a source of complaint. We have all heard the song "Dry Bone" - "the thigh bone connected to the back bone; the back bone connected to the neck bone; the neck bone connected to the head boneS" It emphasizes how everything we do can have an effect on other parts of the body. In my case, with my cervical fusions and the graft from my hip bone, my hip bone is literally connected to the vertebral column.

When a woman gets pregnant, it is the beginning of what I consider to be the greatest creation on the planet. For a moment give some thought to how a child is born with every part intact and in working order. The vertebral column, so intricately created, as are all body parts, will in my opinion challenge forever the science of the current high-tech revolution. How, I wonder, can such a mechanism as vertebrae be created so perfectly? How can such a series of bones be stacked on top of each other, and so aligned as to have a canal through it protecting the spinal cord? Many of us know individuals, or have heard of someone, who has become a para or quadriplegic due to an accident. Our skeletal makeup is a marvel, and it is sad how often we see this body of ours mistreated, and yet we wonder why it is not functioning at peak performance. Wear and tear can come in many forms; it is up to us to have problems attended to at the earliest onset. Our backbone cannot be taken for granted, nor can any other part of the body.

Cervical Vertebrae

Anterior tubercle
Body
Transverse process
Sulcus for spinal nerve
Transverse foramen
Pedicle
Superior articular facet
Costo-transverse bar
Vertebral foramen
Lamina
Spinous process
Inferior articular process
Body
Anterior tubercle
Posterior tubercle

4th cervical vertebra (superior view)

7th cervical vertebra (superior view)

C2
C3
C4
C5
C6
C7
T1

C3
C4
C5

3rd, 4th, and 5th cervical vertebrae (anterior view)

2nd cervical to 1st thoracic vertebrae (right lateral view)

The upper end of the vertebral column (backbone). In my case, the 4/5; 5/6; 6/7 levels were fused together. At the 4/5, and 6/7 levels there was no disk matter left. My vertebrae were bone on bone. At the five six level, it was moderately healthy, but required fusing to stabilize the area.

A myelogram procedure can have some side effects. In my case it was a disaster. It turned out I was allergic to the iodine dye used in the procedure and my reaction to the dye nearly did me in. (A word of advice: If you ever have to have an exploratory investigation involving dyes, find out in advance if there are any alternatives or a choice of dyes that can cause fewer side effects or less of an allergic reaction.)

The procedure took place on a Friday. I was warned that I might have some discomfort or nausea over the weekend but that I would be able to go to work on Monday. This was important as I had been scheduled to testify at an Examination for Discovery on a company-related insurance claim on Monday.

At the beginning of the Examination for Discovery I told those who were involved that I was not feeling all that well but that I would do my duty as best I could. I made it through the morning but by early afternoon I was slipping fast. Since I had finished my testimony by this time, I said that I was going to leave and drive home. What I did not know was how I appeared to those present. My colleagues told me I was not to drive home. They would call a cab and I had to agree to go directly home by cab. By now I was getting sick to my stomach. I had to ask the cab driver to stop the car on three occasions as I did not want to get his car dirtier than I already had. When he delivered me to my home, he actually charged extra for having to clean the car.

I "progressed" from vomiting to splitting headaches to a total loss of balance and ended up at the hospital for a ten-day stay. In addition to all of this, my body turned crimson red with a rash. I could not believe what was happening – and all I had done was find out whether there was a problem in my cervical spine. I was drinking more liquids than I ever had before in an attempt to flush the dye out of my system, and I was bathing in baking soda, which helped to reduce the itching. This episode took me off my feet for a month.

When you find yourself in a painful and dangerous situation like this, you can respond in one of two ways: you can run from it or you can stay and face it and fight it. This is the "Fight or Flight" response. In my case, I was in extreme distress from a split-second incident. I had not had a good day since the accident, and my diary lists a steady stream of medical appointments of one kind or another. I could have run from the pain by taking massive amounts of drugs to deaden the pain and myself. Instead, I felt I had no choice but to stay positive and keep fighting for my health, charting the unknown waters. I had to have a profound belief in myself and in my doctors to deal with problems I had never faced before and believe I was going to overcome them.

As well, I had made a serious and irrevocable commitment to improving my health. Now my health and wellbeing were threatened by an event outside my control. I knew since the day of the accident that something serious had happened to me. My friends, family, and colleagues could see that I was not myself, but none of the doctors or therapists could tell me what was happening to me. All they could suggest was that things might settle in time. If that didn't happen, surgery might be necessary as a last resort.

I decided that in spite of this serious problem I would not abandon my Commitment to Health program. I had been assured that walking would not harm me and could, in fact, be helpful. Flight from my aerobic walking would not stop the pain, so I was determined to continue walking. This was a positive decision as the walking made me feel good and I was making progress. I continued to lose weight, my blood pressure was coming down (from 210/110 to 140/70), and before I knew it I was off blood pressure medication. I was sure it would be regressive to abandon my aerobic walking program. Needless to say, my personal physician was extremely happy with this aspect of my health and my commitment to walking was stronger than ever.

A brief introduction to the spine

At this point, I believe it's important for readers to be conversant in layperson's terms with the spine. I don't want to get technical, but it is important to understand that our vertebrae and the discs in between them play a crucial role in our well being and skeletal function.

The spine is made up of twenty-four bony blocks, the vertebrae, which are piled on top of one another. The spine is divided into five sections – the cervical (neck) region, thoracic (chest), lumbar (lower back), sacral, and coccygeal (tailbone).

The spine is nerve central in the body. The spinal cord runs up the spine to the brain, threading through holes in the centre of each vertebra. From this cord, nerves branch out to all parts of our body.

These nerves carry impulses from the brain throughout our body and back to the brain.

Each vertebra in the spine is separated from the one below by a disc. These discs are made up of a soft jelly-like substance surrounded by a tough outer skin. Discs absorb the shock of all our movement, from the jolts of walking to the strains of turning our head. They keep the vertebrae from rubbing on each other. Without the discs, the spine would be absolutely rigid. The disc can withstand considerable stress and compression and will not slip out from between two vertebrae. Instead, a disc can rupture or herniate, causing the jelly-like substance to expand outside the disc and possibly press against a nerve. If a ruptured disc in the cervical region puts pressure on a nerve it can cause pain and numbness in the arm.

Facet joints are the bones that join two adjacent vertebrae. They are at the back of the vertebrae and act the same way other body joints do, such as the knee joint, allowing a certain range of movement. They let the vertebrae move on each other. Ligaments keep the vertebrae in good alignment and also cushion the shock of excessive movement. Back and abdominal muscles also help to stabilize the spine and absorb jolts and movement. If facet joints, ligaments, or muscles are strained, they can cause back pain.

The cervical spine is where I had my problems. It is composed of seven vertebrae and can move forward (flexion) or backward (extension) and can rotate or bend from one side to the other. In the event of a car accident, however, it can be jolted too far forward or backward (hyperflexion and hyperextension). This can result in soft tissue damage – damage to the muscles and ligaments that have been stretched beyond their capacity or even torn. It can take up to a year or more to fully recover from soft tissue damage.

Degenerative disc disease, which I had as an asymptomatic condition before the accident, can be caused by osteoarthritis of the facet joints, possibly in combination with simple wear and tear on the discs and/or the growth of bone spurs on the vertebra. Pain is caused by the degeneration of the disc, by accompanying muscle spasms and stiffness, and by pressure on nerves as the scarring and tissue build-up of osteoarthritis narrow the space through which the nerves exit or enter the spinal column. According to orthopaedic surgeons D.J.

34

Ogilvie-Harris and G.J. Lloyd in their book *Personal Injury*, "[Recent studies show] quite clearly that in patients with pre-existing degenerative disc disease the incidence of disc disruption and nerve root compression is significantly higher and that recovery after acceleration-deceleration injuries is significantly slower."

Information from:

Workers' Compensation Board of BC. *Back Talk: An Owner's Manual for Backs*. (no city: Workers' Compensation Board, 1987)

Tepperman, Dr. Perry S. M.D. and Frank Roberts. *Sit Up, and Take Care of Your Back*. Vol. 2. (Toronto, ON: OBUSFORME Ltd., 1993)

Ogilvie-Harris, D.J. and G.J. Lloyd. *Personal Injury: A Medico-Legal Guide to the Spine and Limbs*. (Aurora, ON: Canada Law Book Inc., 1986)

Berkow, Robert, M.D. editor-in-chief. *The Merck Manual*. 14th edition. (Rahway, NJ: Merck Sharp & Dohme Research Laboratories, 1982)

Chapter 2

VITAL SIGNS

When a child is born, a quick assessment is made of its organs and vital signs, one of which is the healthy cry of a baby. We are all aware of the joys of a healthy newborn. Certainly Sasha and I were blessed to see our six children born with all vital signs and all vital parts.

It may seem strange to start a chapter in this manner, but vital signs are something we are all born with and have for the rest of our lives. And I personally had taken all of the so-called vital signs for granted.

Over the years as we grow up, we naturally expect our bodies to perform whatever tasks we ask of them. We are subjected to all kinds and levels of stress depending on our activities. How often do we question whether the various nerve centres are going to perform properly for a given activity?

Since my accident I've learned that we actually peak in early life, and our bodies start to degenerate at what may seem like a young age. All too often we take our bodies for granted – until we have a medical checkup and find that there is something amiss in one or more of the vital signs. This may be due to any number of stresses that we have been subjecting our body to, and we are quite taken aback if we are let down. We do not hear of the many breakdowns relating to the public at large, but if we look at sports as an example, there are names and stories in the news on a daily basis.

In my case, a split-second accident had affected me so I could no longer count on my body for anything. Before the accident I had never encountered a health problem that lasted so long or presented so many restrictions. I had to guard against too much head movement, which caused more pain. If I wanted to turn my head I had to turn from the shoulders. Though I continued to attend to my work at the office, it was extremely stressful. The skull pain increased each day and tested my ability to carry on. It's one thing to have a physical presence at the office but quite another to be there mentally when you are fighting a debilitating illness that limits your brain activities because of indescribable pain. Only someone who has experienced such a trauma can know what I am talking about.

Although it was hard to think of myself as disabled, that is exactly what I was. There was no activity – eating a meal, shaving, reading, watching TV, sitting at a desk, driving – that did not cause increased pain. I could no longer participate in games of tennis or bowling, in ice-skating, cross-country skiing, swimming, or cycling – all activities I had enjoyed before the accident. Taking in a movie was a chore as I could not sit through a show without searing pain. I had to give up many activities that were important to me. For example, within the life insurance industry there is a degree – Chartered Life Underwriter (CLU) – that signifies professional competence in the field. Graduates of the intensive five-year course of study can volunteer to lead CLU courses and help further the education of others. I had been conducting courses every week through the fall and winter, and now I carried on with my teaching in spite of the extreme pain. Only the soul knows how difficult a time it was. I ultimately had to give up this activity as well as the hockey and lacrosse coaching that I had been involved with since our sons were participants.

However, in spite of the pain compounded with every step, my Commitment to Health and my walking program remained intact. It is difficult enough to start and maintain an exercise program when you are well; when you are not well it is a battle to continue, but it was a discipline and a goal that kept me going.

I kept thinking of the saying "If it's not broken, don't fix it." My case was the opposite. Nothing was literally broken, but I was convinced I had a major problem that needed to be fixed, a hidden disability. You cannot see a pinched nerve or touch it, but can you ever feel it. I saw myself in the ranks of the walking dead, if there is such a thing, and I could not help but wonder why, with all this medical technology, the doctors could not fix me up. Could a pinched nerve alone cause so much distress? And was there really nothing that could be done about it?

After the myelogram in early 1987, two and a half years after the accident, my orthopaedic surgeon told me that I should have surgery. Specifically, I needed a spinal fusion at the C4/5 level where the nerve was being pinched. There was also some degeneration at the C6/7 disc and the possibility of problems at the C5/6 level.

At this point Dr. McNeill asked me what I thought was a peculiar question. "Jerry," he said, "I do believe you have a structural problem that needs to be surgically corrected. However, I need you to confirm something for me. You do have the pain that you have been describing to me?"

"Stu," I replied, "if I did not have the type of pain I am enduring, I would not be sitting here in your office." I asked him why, at this stage, he was posing such a question.

His response was that in many cases doctors have a problem identifying whether or not corrective surgery is the answer. He said he firmly believed that it was the answer in my case, but he needed that final verbal commitment from me. He told me there was nothing more disturbing than to discover once an operation was underway that the surgery was not necessary.

At this interview Dr. McNeill also warned us that there was always the danger of something going wrong in the procedure I was to undergo. It was his duty to advise us of both the upside and the downside. On the upside, if all went well the pinched nerve would be taken care of and the other two levels would not cause further problems. The downside was that I could come out of surgery a quadri- or paraplegic.

Suddenly I was facing not one fusion but three, as well as the possibility of something going wrong. Sasha and I were no doubt noticeably devastated. The surgeon advised us to go home and think about it, though I knew there was not much to think about as we were dealing with the last resort.

We had a follow-up meeting with the surgeon and he told us that after studying the X-rays again he had decided that surgery should be performed at the C4/5 level, where the nerve was being pinched, but that we should take a wait-and-see approach to the other two levels – fix the obvious and see if the other two levels stabilized without surgery. Dr. McNeill told me that a single fusion had a lower risk factor than doing three fusions at one time, although even one fusion was risky. He also said that he was not optimistic my problem would be fully resolved by a single fusion.

At this visit I asked Dr. McNeill, "Would I have had these problems if the accident had not occurred?" His opinion was that had it not been for the accident, I would probably have lived a normal life without problems. Disc deterioration was taking place unbeknownst to me before the accident, but it was accelerated and worsened by the force of the impact.

I went into Lions Gate Hospital on June 31, 1987, the day before surgery, and the reality of what I was to undergo quickly set in as I was visited by the anaesthetist, a neurologist, and my surgeon. I was told to shower in the evening as well as first thing in the morning before surgery. I remember so vividly the tremendous support I was getting from my wife, even though she too had been worn down by the worry and stress of my problems for the past two and a half years.

I'd never needed surgery before, so had never been in an operating room. I found this in itself to be traumatic – there was a long ride down various corridors, then I was lined up on a stretcher and a number of nurses came by to verify who I was and make sure they were not bringing the wrong person into the operating room. It was a model of precision.

The operating room with all the paraphernalia laid out was a cold, stark setting, not at all welcoming. I looked to my left and there were my X-rays and my surgeon discussing his strategy with my personal physician. It was not long after my arrival in the operating room that the anaesthetist did his job and I knew no more until I returned to consciousness some time later in the recovery room. As I emerged from the anaesthetic, I found a nurse holding me down. I was trying to get up and waving my hands desperately.

Briefly, the operation I underwent begins with an incision in the throat area. From there the surgeon works his way to the front of the two vertebrae to be fused. He removes the disc matter between them and chisels an opening in each of the vertebrae (see diagram), then goes to the hip area and chisels out a piece of hip bone to insert into the opening in the vertebrae. He inserts this bone and presto! you have what is referred to as a cervical fusion. This piece of bone holding your vertebrae apart plays an important part in your anatomy for the rest of your life. (My short explanation does not do justice to the skills of the surgeon who devoted so much time to such a specialized area of medical practice.)

Anterior Interbody Fusion by Dowel Graft

In the text, I briefly discuss the cervical surgical procedure ending with the words "presto! you have what is referred to as a cervical fusion." If only it were that easy!

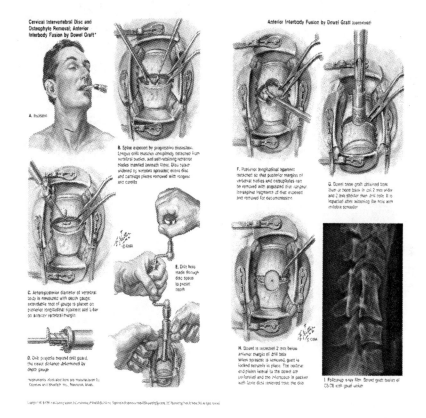

The illustration shows the detailed step-by-step procedure which medical technology has perfected.

41

Anterior Cervical Fusion - Cloward Procedure

Anterior Cervical Fusion - Cloward Procedure

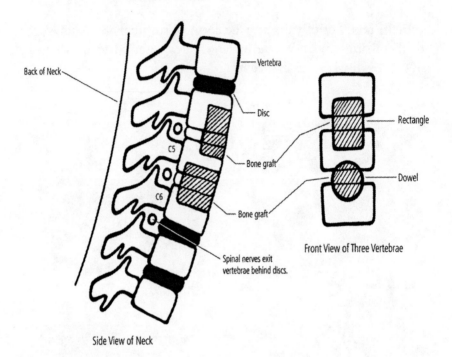

Side View of Neck

Front View of Three Vertebrae

Cloward Procedure -

-- Removal of disc and bone spurs
-- Drill hole involving two adjacent vertebrae C5, and C6
-- Insert bone dowel into drill hole
-- Note alternative use of rectangular trough and bone graft.

Illustration by Dr. Stuart R. McNeil, M.D., B.A., F.R.C.S. (C)

In this illustration Dr. McNeil shows two types of graft. In my case it required three procedures as shown in the prior illustration, with the use of a rectangular trough and bone graft taken from my hip area.

After surgery, my vital signs were continually being monitored. I was asked literally every hour each day to move each and every part of my body. The nurses carefully monitored the results. The routine was so precise that I was able to anticipate the request for the next movement. Occasionally the nurse giving the test would outsmart me by asking for a non-routine movement or by rearranging the order of requests.

After I came out of the anaesthetic I had a tingling in three fingers on both hands. This became the focal point of every vital sign review. A number of doctors came in to see me and discuss this tingling in the fingers. A neurologist gave me an extensive examination. After a few days of this I became concerned, as everybody coming in to see me was asking about the tingling in my fingers. It seemed like the surgery was secondary or had failed somehow, but it had in fact been successful. The tingling was caused by nerves irritated or damaged during the surgery.

We take for granted our control of our body. I was to learn, as time went by, that no matter what I did or how hard I tried, there was absolutely nothing I could do about this tingling. My body had control over me. The sensation is one that most everyone has felt at one time or another when a part of your body has "gone to sleep" and gives you a tingling sensation when you try to wake it up. In my case, this tingling goes on continually.

After twelve days in the hospital I was up and around, walking the halls with my cane, trying to get in as much walking as possible, although I was extremely slow. The greatest pain came from the stitches in my hip area. After surgery I wore the cervical collar, which I slept and wept in for the months to come. It was summertime and our home was located high above the city on the mountainside, a good location for rest and recovery.

Prior to surgery my doctors had told me I would have to take three months off work. This was hard to accept, especially since I had never lost a day's work due to illness in over twenty-two years prior to the accident. Nevertheless, I told myself that three months was a small price to pay to get well and back to work.

My company was most understanding, having both my and its own interests in mind. It brought in an acting manager to run the office during my absence. This provided me with peace of mind. I knew that with the help of head office there would be an element of order and control. Obviously you cannot bring in a replacement and expect to have textbook performance based on your own standards, but my replacement knew he was under scrutiny for a future promotion and he did as well as he could under the circumstances.

We all have a lot to learn about disability and recuperation. I learned that after major surgery you do not spend time with your stand-in, getting him set up, especially when you have been home from the hospital only a few days. I paid the price but had the satisfaction of knowing I had done as much as I could for the stranger who was running my office for me. Over the coming months our contact was kept to a minimum for obvious reasons; the acting manager worked with a contact person in head office as much as possible.

A major development during this crisis management period was a discussion with head office that led to a decision that I should hire an assistant manager on a permanent basis. This individual would be my support person when I returned to the office. He or she would help me with the work when I got back, as I could not be expected to function at maximum performance immediately. We had been discussing such an expansion prior to my surgery, so I had a short list of candidates already.

Here I was recuperating from major surgery, and a vice president was willing to fly out and assist me in interviewing candidates if I would line them up. I was supposed to be resting and relaxing, and I was indeed flat on my back in bed. But I was flat on my back making phone calls to potential candidates and arranging for interviews at our home on two separate days. I must have been out of my mind to agree to such an arrangement, and had my surgeon known of this he would probably have insisted that I stop.

The interviews went well, my medication held me together, and we came up with a candidate to whom I offered the position. Now I had an acting manager who was to stay until I returned to work and an assistant manager who would settle into his position and help me when I returned.

In retrospect, carrying a workload like this was not conducive to my recovery, especially since I had been given strict orders to stay away from my office. That certainly did not mean bringing it home to my bedroom. However, I believed that anyone loyal and dedicated would do the same thing as long as they were able and could get away with it. At the time it seemed easier to deal with the crisis and get the job done. But at what price to my health?

Now I have learned that rest and relaxation must be a priority. Personal vital signs are more important than the vital signs of a business, especially since the business procedures we have established will usually continue to run smoothly without us.

I remember a former major in the Canadian Armed Services who I met while I was in high school. He told me the story of his career, which left a lasting impression on me as he was still bitter about it even years after it ended. He said that he had come up through the ranks and was thoroughly enjoying his career. It was a great surprise to him when he was told that there was no longer a need for his services. As he put it, "Here I was a number of years away from retirement and suddenly without a job." He emphasized how he had felt he was an important cog in the service. Then he said, "I found out that I was not indispensable." He went on and on about how he felt no one could move into his secure position. But they did move in while he moved out. I believe that his words were with me at the time of my convalescence. In my case, the job was waiting for me; what I needed was my health.

My progress at home was favourable. I continued my daily walks, receiving a lot of sympathy from our neighbours who would stop and talk to me. I was often walking with a family member, as our children and grandchildren were coming and going throughout the summer. When I was not in bed resting, I was at poolside, watching the grandchildren learn their swimming and diving skills. All of them learned to retrieve silver coins and loonies from the bottom of the pool.

X-rays showed I was healing nicely and after two months of confinement I was told I could start taking short outings as part of the recuperative process. It was great to get into a car again, especially, after a few outings, into the driver's seat.

By the end of August I was on top of the world. My blood pressure readings were 140 over 70 (down from 210 over 110 since I started my aerobic walking program) and I was fully expecting that when I saw the surgeon again in mid-September, he would okay my return to work.

I had an appointment with my personal physician in late August, and he commented on how well I looked and how pleased my surgeon would be when he saw me. Dr. B was happy with my ongoing Commitment to Health program. My weight loss and lowered blood pressure showed that the daily walk was doing me a lot of good in spite of the fact I was recuperating from major surgery. The doctor added that in the next two weeks I should start removing the cervical collar for an hour a day.

I had been in the collar since before my surgery, so this was welcome news. As instructed, I started to remove the collar for an hour each day. On the first day it seemed strange to be without the collar, and the strangeness continued every day for the next four days. However, by the end of the first week I was telling Sasha about a strange skull pain. It could be a headache, but it was unlike anything I had ever experienced.

I continued removing the collar, and by the time I saw the surgeon a week later I had skull pain so bad I wanted to tear my hair out. It felt like my head was in a vise. I was in unbearable pain and all I could do was plead for help. The turnaround in my health was most devastating considering I had been in such good health only two weeks before.

Dr. McNeill was pleased to hear about the progress I had made prior to taking the collar off, but he did not advise me to start using the collar again. He said it was important that I keep it off for the better part of the day. At the same time, he could see the distress I was in and immediately made arrangements for me to see a neurologist that very day.

Chapter 3

HORROR STORY

Dr. Shirley Baker-Thomas, the neurologist, had previously attended to me when I was in the hospital with the severe myelogram reaction, so it was not as if I were seeing someone for the first time. She remembered me well and was sympathetic about my obvious decline in health. She noted that my blood pressure was back in the 220/110 range when only two weeks earlier it had been 140/70. However, two weeks earlier I had not been suffering excruciating skull pain.

Neurologically, all visual findings were favourable so she put me on medication to take care of the elevated blood pressure, ordered a CAT scan, and told me to go home and rest. Dr. Baker-Thomas requested the CAT scan as a precaution, to see if some new or overlooked condition had developed. A CAT scan (CAT stands for computerized axial tomography) is a computerized image – in my case, of the skull – that will show if there is bleeding, a tumour, or other problems. The scan showed nothing and the skull pains were barely affected by the medication. It was obvious that I was not ready to remove the collar.

I entered a program of physiotherapy at Lions Gate Hospital and the physiotherapists had me start wearing the cervical collar again in the hopes of getting me back to where I had been at the end of August. I received no relief from wearing the collar, so we decided that I should quit using it as it would have to come off at some point in any event. The physio treatment was also unsuccessful and the surgeon stopped it. I was not ready for any type of massage or manipulation.

By now it was October 1987 and I still had vise-gripping skull pain, medication was giving me little relief, my hands were tingling, and I was a month past my due date for returning to work.

The major concern was to pinpoint where all the pain was coming from. It seemed to begin in the neck area and radiate to the skull, and any head movement produced compounded pain. Dr. McNeill suggested that my problem could be psychological, comparing it to the cases of patients who continue to feel pain after surgery, amputation of a limb, etc. This didn't take into account the fact that up until the time the collar started coming off I was a walking specimen of good health with no pain whatsoever.

Dr. McNeill agreed and said the two unfused vertebrae levels might be the underlying cause of my pain, but he could leave no stone unturned. All he had to go on was X-rays and the myelogram. These showed there was some kind of problem with the discs, but could he be sure this was the cause of my ongoing pain? Until he operated and saw the site for himself, he couldn't determine how bad it was, but he still feared doing unnecessary surgery. I knew I put him in a difficult position. Here I was seeking medical help and he had to decide the precise nature of that help without exposing me to undue risk. I knew he was doing his utmost to help me.

In late October I talked to the surgeon about going back to work. If I was just going to lie around at home with a big headache, wouldn't it be logical for me to try returning to work, if only for a few hours a day? Maybe with time I could work myself out of this mess. After all, the surgery had been successful. In retrospect, I see that this was a workaholic's way of getting around things. My surgeon's reply was it was okay with him if I could get away with it.

I do not know why this gave me a sense of relief, as it did nothing to decrease my pain. On the other hand, I felt I had gained something. The surgeon had certainly not given me a clean bill of health – how could he when I was in his office screaming for help? – but all I was looking for was an escape in the hope that a new environment might be the answer.

In any event, I returned to work, going in daily. And frankly, by the time I got to the office I was already in such compounded pain that I should have immediately gone home. But no, I was willing to subject myself to even more punishment in an attempt to work the problem out of the system.

Months went by. A number of times I went in to see doctors at the local hospital's emergency room. Dr. McNeill also sent me to a surgeon specializing in internal medicine. Now I see he was following the process of elimination. He had to get to the root of my problem, ensure it was not neurological, internal, psychological, or mechanical. The internist would also confirm there was no secondary problem developing.

When I saw this specialist I found his questioning was thorough, concerned with my home life, my work, any financial difficulties, my marital relationship, and any outstanding insurance claim. He performed an exhaustive examination, found I was in good health, prescribed some new medication that he hoped would break the cycle of pain, and sent me on my way, wishing my wife and I the best. He assured me he would write a report to my surgeon as well as my personal physician. He did write a lengthy report, but nothing had changed.

The new medication did not work so in desperation I dropped in on my personal physician. Dr. B suggested that I try doubling up on the medication. This gave me some marginal relief but at a high cost. I felt continually spaced out, with pain only slightly subdued. It is the emptiest of feelings to be overwrought by pain while knowing that nobody can help you. I had always felt that there was an answer or treatment for most medical problems. I was in total agony from day to day, feeling helpless and wondering what was going on and what was happening to me. My hours at the office were largely non-productive, but it was a place to go. Although I did attend to some matters, it was painful doing any work.

In March 1988 my personal physician asked me if I should perhaps try the cervical collar again. I told him that out of desperation, frustration, and nowhere else to turn I had worn the collar on the weekend and received slight relief. So slight and yet it was wonderful compared to the extreme discomfort I felt the rest of the time. We agreed I should give the collar a try and report to the surgeon on the results.

Simultaneously, Dr. B arranged for me to see a high-priced neurological consultant, one of the big boys in the big league, for an assessment. I accepted the statement at face value. At this point I was vulnerable to any suggestion and my only question was, "Why are you sending me to another neurologist? The last one did not seem to have any answers other than to prescribe some medication for elevated blood pressure due to the high stress I was experiencing."

His response was that this was one of the top neurologists and we should hear what he had to say. On arriving at the appointed time I had to wait a short while before the neurologist came out, introduced himself, and asked me to come into his office. He was an elderly gentleman so my initial thought was, "Well here I am with age and experience. It will be interesting to see what he comes up with."

His questioning was thorough and precise as he reviewed my file, which he had in front of him and which had been sent for his perusal by my personal physician. He also moved like lightning from one subject to another. When he asked me why I had my cervical collar on, who had instructed me to wear it, and told me that I should not have worn it for more than a few days after surgery, I began to wonder why I was in his office. He was openly criticizing the medical care I had been receiving. Was I here to get a neurological opinion or to have holes torn in my personal physician's records? Apprehension was setting in as I had never had this type of examination before.

When he started to question me about the insurance corporation involved in my claim regarding the accident that precipitated my problem, I really began to wonder what I was doing there. Then he wondered aloud how he could relate my problem to an accident that had occurred years earlier. It suddenly dawned on me that perhaps I had been sent to this doctor at the insurance corporation's request for an independent report and that my personal physician had decided not to tell me this reason.

The interview continued, an interrogation of Dr. B's files. He raised no questions of his own. After a lengthy questioning period he asked me to step into his examining room. Before I knew it he had thrown my head around four ways and pounded his fist down my back. I saw stars in my eyes.

He stated that seeing as I was driving I should wear the cervical collar home, but I should take it off as soon as I got home and keep it off. I repeated that I had just started wearing it again in the last few days and that it was giving me some relief, but he completely ignored my statement and ordered me to follow his advice.

I left his office in a daze, shaking, and arrived home in a disturbed state. I was devastated by such an unprofessional examination and disillusioned by the fact I had gone to see him in the first place.

I went to see my personal physician soon after this examination, both to ask him about wearing the cervical collar and to show him the bruises left on my lower back by the fist pounding. Dr. B's comment was, "He really killed you."

My surgeon was appalled when I described the neurologist's examination. He said, "It was a strange examination," and ordered some X-rays of my back.

In his written report the neurologist stated that I was suffering "post-traumatic neurosis" and "rather than medication for hypertension [he] recommended an anti-depressant."

I still question the value of the verbal interview and the physical examination and wonder what was accomplished. I was prepared to lay a complaint with the College of Physicians and Surgeons, but I could not disagree when friends and colleagues told me that I already had enough on my plate. For a long time after that examination I would on occasion wake up in a cold sweat, reliving the experience.

Writing for survival

How do you retain your faith and keep your spirits up through this kind of a medical ordeal? I cannot overstate the peace of mind and therapeutic effect I realized by keeping a diary. It gave me an uplift with every entry, whether it was positive or negative. The positives were constant reinforcement, giving me the inner strength to carry on. The negatives allowed me a daily release of frustrations and gave me a sense of relief. By diarizing the negatives, even when they became repetitive, I handled them as they came up. By writing them in my diary I put them out of my mind and eliminated a lot of negative self-talk, always a trouble spot.

And who else could I have dumped this on? My wife had a full-time job caring for me. On occasion she would read what I had written on a given day and as she read, tears would flow. I tried to share as many positives as I could with Sasha, but as far as negatives were concerned she only had to look at me and she could observe the negatives. As much as I would have liked to, I often could not cover up how bad I was feeling on a given day.

What friend could I call daily for months and years to tell what I had gone through the previous day? Who would want to listen, who would understand, and how could they help? Sasha and I agreed that when family or friends came over I would not use them as a dumping ground, but sometimes this happened anyway because of an interesting question that could not be answered with a yes or no. The daily entry required no response.

I do not know if I could call my appointments with doctors a dumping ground. I certainly told them what was bothering me, but what I was looking for from them was help to solve my medical problem. In my particular case, when my self-talk revolved about my medical problem I would write down any questions that came up so I could discuss them with the appropriate medical practitioner. In the initial stages, when I was relying on self-talk and memory, I would forget the questions I wanted to ask. I had not just one question but a multitude, and how could I remember one or many when I was not only not well but was so heavily medicated that I was walking around like a zombie? Preparing written notes on what I wanted to cover was quick, thorough, and never left me wondering whether I had asked all the questions I wanted to. I urge anyone who is seeing medical practitioners to write out questions you want to review on your next visit and every visit thereafter. This also expedites the visits, as you can be sure you will cover areas of concern to you. If you are able to communicate but unable to do your own writing, I urge your caregiver to do it for you. It will make life easier for all concerned.

All my entries were in a scribbler, dated, with three or four words on the weather and then the time of day noted. Sometimes there would be a short paragraph, a page, or occasionally a couple of pages. Usually I would first write about the significance of the past twenty-four hours. Then, often, the notes would be more wide-ranging. I would reflect on whatever came to mind, sometimes wandering off well into the past. The entries kept me more closely aware of my condition, and whenever there were some positives to put down on paper it was such great encouragement, reinforcing my thoughts and feelings.

I do not believe that the thoughts and questions I wrote simply occurred to me at the moment of writing. I am sure that many of the things I put to paper were the result of my subconscious working. When I did my daily notes, I was never lacking for something to write. What I found was that, having related the events and thoughts of the previous day, the thought processes would carry on and I would have a page or two written in what seemed like no time at all. I would let the thoughts flow.

I found it fascinating that just as my walking had become part of my daily routine, so did my writing. Although this activity only took a few minutes of my day, putting my thoughts to paper took away a lot of the negative self-talk that would no doubt have been building up until it grew into a monstrous snowball. By dealing with a small snowball daily, there was a daily meltdown. It felt good.

I should emphasize that you do not need to force yourself to find positive things to write in a diary. If all you are feeling one day is negative, write that down. It does not matter how positive or negative the notes are on any given day. What matters is that you write an entry. Get whatever you have to say off your chest.

If you are enduring problems of any type whatsoever, I urge you to get a scribbler and start keeping a daily diary. Say it the way you feel it on the day with no corrections, additions, or deletions in hindsight. It may be difficult at first – it was hard for me in the beginning – but do as much as you can. If there are many negatives, get them all out in writing.

Do not worry about how much you write. If you can write many pages on your first day, do so. Write for as long as you can. And if it is only a few lines, there is nothing wrong with that. You may want to write a few lines at a time, finishing an entry gradually over the day. Start writing and just keep adding to it whenever thoughts occur to you. Do not leave a thought unwritten in hopes that you will remember it the next day. As well, it is important to start fresh every day. Put all the good, bad, and indifferent to paper on the day it occurs and start your next day with a new page.

Originally I wrote my entries late in the day, but as time went on I began to do them first thing in the morning after my daily walk and breakfast. When I was in business, this was when I did my serious detail work, when I found myself to be sharpest. I found this earlier time allowed me to reflect on the previous day and on how I was feeling now compared to the day before. I also found that when I started making my entries in the morning, the thoughts flowed better. Writing in the evening tended to be more of a chore. As I was thinking about the day, the thoughts were full of negatives – not the best way to end a day. Moreover, why leave it to the end of the day? I had twenty-four hours a day to do what I could.

Even if you do not have serious health problems, a daily diary can help you explore and clarify problems and decisions you are facing. If you are a caregiver, working closely with someone in pain or with a disability, and can relate to what I have said, take the time to help the individual you care for start a diary, writing down the daily notes if the person in your care cannot do it.

Every human being is burdened with ongoing problems. In spite of these, most of us continue to hold on and try not to give up. As we face our problems, mulling them over in our heads, we use self-talk to dwell on the positive and the negative aspects and our choices. We are often torn between the right and wrong decision. This is the natural thing to do: if I have a problem, I deal with it and get it out of the way. This is healthy. However, because of our ability to rationalize, I believe that we often overrule the positive and hang on to the negative self-talk.

By writing out my progress, worries, thoughts, and activities, I would end up feeling good every day. Deep down I felt I had a mission. I was determined that one day, God willing, I would tell my story. Had I not been keeping a diary, I would not have had the recall of events I do. Once I made an entry, I never reread it until I came to write this book. As I reread the entries I recalled the events, the pain I was in, and, later, the progress that was giving me a new lease on life. The release I felt writing it down and the hope I feel writing this book show for me the power of pen and paper.

Chapter 4

MASSAGE AND MANIPULATION

When I saw Dr. McNeill in early 1988, he was pleased to hear that I was receiving some relief by wearing the cervical collar. Up until now I had been using a soft collar, but now we decided to try a more rigid type of support.

I was fitted with what is called a Philadelphia collar. The Philadelphia collar was like a cast. It rested on my shoulders and held my head in one place. I could not turn my head without turning my whole upper body. This collar gave me more support through the neck area, as well as providing a place for my chin to rest. It was quite uncomfortable, especially in the summer when it was often hot and itchy, but it did provide me with some relief and my surgeon decided that we should again try a light physio and massage program.

In April 1988, at the beginning of this course of treatment, the physiotherapist found my muscles were tense and I was extremely sensitive to touch in the neck area. We tried many types of physiotherapy, from hot packs and cold packs to massage as well as an isotonic and isometric exercise program. Isotonic exercises involve movement and contraction – turning my head, tucking my chin, shrugging my shoulders – to improve neck mobility. Isometric exercises use contraction without movement to increase strength (see the examples of isotonic and isometric exercises at the end of this chapter). When I started the exercise program I could not move my head in any direction without suffering compounded pain. As the physio visits continued, my blood pressure began to rise again. The increasing pain and stress was taking its toll and my body was telling me so. I was also beginning to have dizzy spells that nearly caused me to pass out. I had never experienced anything like this before and it was scary.

After three months and nineteen physiotherapy visits I was definitely in worse shape than I had been when I started the program.

It had gotten to the point where the physiotherapist could not lay a hand on me anywhere in the neck area as I was so tender.

Immediately after my accident I had not responded to physiotherapy. After my surgery I did not respond to physiotherapy. Now another round of physiotherapy had to be aborted because it was only making my condition worse. This had been the longest and most extensive program to date. Every form of manipulation had been tried, with no success. I was a willing patient but my body was not willing to respond. I had been to see a neurologist, an internist, and yet another physiotherapist, with no solution in sight. It seemed obvious to me that this was a problem only surgery could alleviate. All other attempts to treat it only aggravated the situation.

However, my personal physician and surgeon still had a lot of questions they wanted answered before another operation: was the problem continued soft tissue injury? Was it caused by muscle atrophy due to the prolonged use of the cervical collar? Was it caused by deterioration at the other two areas of my spine that the surgeon had recognized as needing fusion? Was it psychological? My medical advisors started to hint that I might need psychiatric help, that perhaps this pain was partially, or all, "in my mind."

As I thought about this suggestion, I found it difficult to see the value of this kind of help when I was feeling so much pain in my neck and skull, compounded by any type of head movement. What was the point of seeing a psychiatrist when I was wearing a cervical neck collar, using a lot of medication, taking a lot of bed rest, and barely getting by on a daily basis? In my mind I knew there was something drastically wrong with my body. Why couldn't that problem be fixed? How would a psychiatrist make any difference to it? I could not help remembering how good I felt after my surgery. I also thought about what had happened when I stopped wearing the cervical collar. Had removing it caused psychological pain? I thought not, and I wondered how a psychiatrist would get to the root of the problem if it were mechanical.

By this time I was stressed out and at my wit's end, wondering why I was not getting relief from the various methods of treatment I had been subjected to. I was as concerned about the amount of medication I was taking as my medical advisors were, especially since it was having little effect and I was told that any more medication would put me flat on my back. I continued to refill my medicine cabinet with painkillers, anti-inflammatories, Inderal, Lasix, Indocid, Fiorinal, blood pressure medication. I was beginning to feel I was a part owner of the local pharmacy.

I must give laurels to the pharmacist who was filling the prescriptions, as she was watchful of both the type and mix of prescriptions I was given. An understanding and interested pharmacist can be a valuable part of your health recovery program. Pharmacists fill prescriptions, but they can also monitor the mix of drugs you are taking and offer valuable assistance, telling you if a combination of drugs might produce unexpected side effects. It is wise to ask questions of the pharmacist if you have the slightest doubt about what you are taking or about to take.

The few hours each day I spent at my insurance office and the time I spent driving were obviously adding to my stress, and there was no relief from pain. Summer was ending and I was no closer to getting better. Instead I was deteriorating and wondering where I should go from there.

On my next visit to the surgeon, he asked whether I had used a TENS device. He explained these devices gave relief to some people. I was all ears as I'd never heard of this before. I would be willing to try anything if it might give me relief, especially if it meant I could get away with using less medication. I got a prescription for the device, purchased it rather than renting, saw a physiotherapist at Lions Gate Hospital who trained me in its placement and use, and was in business.

The TENS device was the size of a TV remote control and attached to my belt or shirt pocket. I could put it on in the morning and carry it with me all day. Wires ran from the device to the back of my neck. Four suction cups were attached to the wires. When these cups were properly placed on my skin I could activate the device to send electric pulses to the trouble spot. These electric impulses relieved the pain both by stimulating my body to produce natural painkillers and by overriding the pain messages sent by my pinched nerves and deteriorating discs with messages that said everything was okay. I could control the amount of current I sent to the pain site. At the high end, the electrical grip from the current was quite strong. I quickly learned that with a high electrical setting I could actually eliminate the pain. It seemed like I had a winner. Instead of going home by eleven a.m., I was extending my day at the office by a few hours.

Unfortunately, I also learned that you do not fool around with your body. You may be able to fool your brain some of the time, but I was trying to fool it on a daily basis and it backfired.

As I was suffering high levels of pain, it took high levels of current to override the pain. By extending my work hours, all I did was leave myself in super-compounded pain by the end of the day. Not only did I need to continue the medication, but I also found that the levels of current I was using were becoming less effective. I immediately stopped using the device and told my surgeon that it had camouflaged the pain, but in doing so it had a regressive effect on me.

More time had passed and I was continuing to tolerate a lot of pain, so much so that I began to wonder how much a human body could endure. I was receiving excellent medical care – every time I dropped in on my personal physician he emphasized how much he wished he could help me, but he too was baffled. I was wearing the hard Philadelphia collar all the time, but was getting worse rather than better.

My surgeon asked me to experiment by using the soft collar for a few hours a day. After interchanging collars for a short while on a daily basis, I quickly found out that I experienced considerably higher levels of pain with the soft collar. As a result of this experiment my surgeon recommended that I have another test.

My first thought was, "How many more tests are there that I have not yet had?" But I did feel a sudden ray of hope that this procedure – magnetic resonance imaging – might help us find out what was causing me so much grief.

Isotonic and isometric exercises

EXCERSIZES FOR THE NECK AND SHOULDERS

ISOMETRIC EXERCISES (contraction with movement for increased mobility)

1. CHIN TURN

Stand or sit erect with chin tucked in close to chest. Turn head slowly to right trying to bring your chin over your right shoulder. Hold for three seconds. Rotate head back to centre position. Pause. Repeat in opposite direction. Repeat entire sequence 5 times.

2. CHIN UP

Push chin downward, trying to touch it to your chest without causing too much strain. Pause. Slowly tilt head backward as far as possible, without straining. Pause. Repeat 5 times. Do not do this exercise if you have CERVICAL ARTHRITIS and avoid extension if it hurts.

3. HEAD TURN

Bend your head slowly to the right trying to bring your right ear to your right shoulder. Pause. Return slowly to centre position. Pause. Repeat in opposite direction. Repeat sequence 5 times.

4. HEAD CIRCLE

Roll your head clockwise in as wide a circle as possible for three complete circles. Do the same in the counter-clockwise direction. Pause. Repeat sequence 3 times. If you have CERVICAL ARTHRITIS modify this exercise so that you only do half circles to the front of the body.

5. SHOULDER SHRUG

Stand erect, arms held loosely at sides. Breathe deeply as you lift your shoulders, first as high, and then as far back as they will move. Breathe out as you lower your shoulders to the starting position and relax. Repeat 20 times, at least twice a day. Build up to 50 times twice a day.

6. UPPER BACK STRETCH

Sit erect. Place hands on shoulders. Try to cross your elbow by bringing your right arm to the left and left arm to the right, until you feel the stretch across your upper back. Return to the starting position, drop your hands and relax. Repeat 10 times.

7. PENDULAR EXERCISE

Hold a 1-2 pound weight in your hand. Bending your knees slightly, bend forward at the waist and hold onto a table with your other hand. Allow your arm to dangle freely (A). Swing your arm laterally across your body to the right and left for 1 minute, keeping your elbow perfectly straight. (B) Then swing your arm backward and forward for 1 minute (C). Now swing your arm in a gradually increasing (clockwise) circle for 1 minute. (D) And finally repeat (C) counterclockwise.

8. CLIMBING-THE-WALL EXERCISE

Face the wall. Keeping your elbows straight, "walk" your fingers up the wall as high as they can go. (Do not shrug or hunch your shoulder. Do not tilt the upper half of your body.) Repeat 10 times, each time trying to "walk" a little higher. Turn your body slightly and repeat 10 times. Continue gradually turning your body and repeating the exercise until you are at a right angle to the wall. Perform the exercise for 10 minutes, 2 or 3 times a day.

ISOMETRIC EXERCISES (contraction without movement for increased strength)

9. RESISTED FLEXION (NECK)

Stand or sit erect. Place your hands on your forehead with one hand on top of the other. Push your head forward against the heel of your hand without moving your head. Hold for a count of 10 (7 seconds). Relax. Repeat 3 times.

10. RESISTED EXTENSION (NECK)

Stand or sit erect. Clasp your hands behind your head – not your neck. Push your head backward against the resisting hands without moving your head. Hold for a count of 10 (7 seconds). Relax. Repeat 3 times.

11. RESISTED SIDE-BEND

Stand or sit erect. Place your right hand on the right side of your face. Push your head sideward against your hand without moving your head. Hold for a count of 10 (7 seconds). Relax. Repeat in opposite direction, with left hand on left temple, etc. Relax. Repeat sequence 3 times.

12. RESISTED ROTATION

Stand or sit erect. Place your right hand on your right temple and your left hand on the left side of the back of your head (your hands should be diagonally opposite). Attempt to look over your right shoulder, resisting the movement of your head with your hands. Hold for a count of 10 (7 seconds). Relax. Repeat in opposite direction with your left hand on your left temple, etc. Relax. Repeat sequence 3 times.

13. RESISTED FLEXION

Stand or sit erect. Raise both forearms in front of your body – parallel to the ground – with your elbows bent. Intertwine your fingers and pull. Hold for a count of 7 (5 seconds). Relax. Repeat 3 times.

14. RESISTED EXTENSION (SHOULDER)

Stand or sit erect. Raise both forearms in front of your body – parallel to the ground – with your elbows bent. Place both palms flat against each other and press. Hold for a count of 7 (5 seconds). Relax. Repeat 3 times.

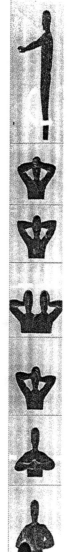

Chapter 5

MAGNETIC RESONANCE IMAGING (MRI)

Dr. McNeill said that the magnetic resonance imaging or MRI test would have to be done at the University of British Columbia Hospital as it was the only place where the necessary equipment was available. He told me he'd contact the hospital directly himself and the hospital would call me to set a time when I could come in for the procedure.

I was anxious to have the MRI done, so I followed up when I hadn't heard from UBC Hospital some two weeks later. After considerable searching the administrator told me that my surgeon's requisition had been misplaced. She was most sympathetic and apologetic for any inconvenience, confirmed with him that it had been sent, and then told me that I was looking at a minimum six-month waiting period once they had the requisition. My heart dropped. Here I was in total distress and now there would be further delay.

I asked the administrator what information she needed before I underwent the procedure and told her I would gather all the necessary documents and hand-deliver the package. Then I asked if the equipment was running continuously.

Yes, she said, and they were fully booked for six months.

Did they ever have a cancellation?

She said that on occasion there would be a cancellation due to unforeseen circumstances. In those cases the equipment sat idle unless, of course, a patient was available on short notice, within two hours.

I told her that I would be available on such short notice and that I would be in with all the required data as soon as we could get it together.

Dr. McNeill was most cooperative, completing a new requisition for the MRI, and we picked this up immediately. Sasha was also extremely supportive. It is incredible how much we come to rely on a caregiver in circumstances like this. She was driving me around most of the time and was busy picking up all the X-rays that had been taken of my neck. Within two days all the homework was done and my wife and I delivered the package personally. The material was checked out and UBC Hospital informed us that they had everything they needed. Moreover, we were advised that because I would be available on short notice, the six-month waiting period could be cut back significantly. I hoped so, as it was now July and six months would take us into the next year.

Well, as the saying goes, take some action and you may have a reaction. Within two weeks, on August 16, 1988, I had a call to come in for an MRI. I was elated.

Time was of the essence, however, as we still had to get to the hospital and it was a long distance from one end of town to the other at a busy time of the day. It turned out it was a good thing that this was our second trip to the hospital complex on the UBC campus, where you can lose a lot of time if you do not know where you are going. We made it with about fifteen minutes to spare, just enough time for the admissions procedure.

Up to this point, all I knew about the MRI was that I would be having some X-rays taken with advanced technology. I was not expecting to be asked what type of music I liked and offered a selection of tapes and a set of earphones. On questioning why I needed taped music, I was led to another room, shown a machine that looked like a tunnel that was closed at both ends, and told that I would be locked in that enclosure for an hour.

I picked out some tapes and went back to the MRI X-ray machine. It had a door at one end. The assistant opened the door, pulled out a cot, and asked me to lie down on it. I was given instructions on how I could have the operator stop the procedure should I get frightened or claustrophobic. Then I was rolled into the tunnel, the door was closed, the music started playing, and within moments I began hearing strange noises. This was the noise of the X-rays being taken. It sounded as if someone was hitting the outer shell of the machine with a fist slowly and then in rapid succession, repeating the process over and over again. I was told there were about twenty-four X-rays taken – these are a series of pictures that are virtual slices of the area of the body being X-rayed. An operator monitored the images on a computer screen as the pictures were taken. As I left the hospital I felt good about this encounter with high technology and was prepared to accept whatever the findings may be, for better or worse.

Shortly after this I had a meeting with my surgeon to discuss the results of the MRI. The radiologist's report said that the MRI showed the discs at the 5/6 and 6/7 levels of my cervical spine, directly below the already-fused 4/5 level, were bulging. The report also said that the nature of the test was beyond the scope of the equipment, something which to this day I have not had explained satisfactorily.

Something that was beyond the scope of my mind was the question of how much of a bulge there was day-to-day. When I was prepared for the MRI I was fitted with a Philadelphia collar that had the effect of stretching my neck. As well, when I was lying down my neck and spine did not have to carry the weight of my skull. How much of a bulge would there have been if I had not been wearing the collar when the X-rays were taken? More to the point, how much of a bulge was there when I was walking around with a collar and the full weight of my skull bearing down on my neck and spine? Little wonder I was feeling continuous pain. At least now I had something definitive that could explain all of the problems I was having.

For my surgeon, the results of the MRI were conclusive. Since I continued to have problems at the 5/6 and 6/7 levels, he said I should consider further surgery. He wanted to discuss my case with a neurosurgeon for a second opinion. This doctor confirmed the MRI findings and agreed that surgery was necessary, though he never saw me personally.

When my personal physician received the results of the MRI, he decided I should have a consultation with yet another neurologist before anything further was attempted. Dr. B wanted this second opinion from Dr. Keyes, a neurologist who did not practise surgery and would stay away from the knife if at all possible.

By now I was not concerned about staying away from the knife; I was determined to get the problem, whatever it was, fixed without any further delay. If there was an organic, structural problem that required repair, I wanted it fixed so I could get on with my life. This continued exposure to procedures and medications that gave me little help made me feel there was still some question that my problem was psychological and surgery might not be necessary. I knew this was not true.

I had to wait several months for an appointment with Dr. Keyes. In the meantime I had been practising many relaxation techniques and also found that I could get some further relief with the Philadelphia collar. By stuffing washcloths under my chin and around the collar I could both hold my neck more firmly in the collar and fractionally stretch my neck. By stretching my neck I was producing a form of traction and taking pressure off the discs. It was most uncomfortable, but the slightest relief was a lot.

Around this time I received a call from Dr. McNeill's secretary who said that my surgeon and my personal physician had decided that I should see yet another doctor with whom they had been working. Dr. Marlene Hunter had been having a high degree of success treating patients with hypnosis.

I found it difficult to understand this suggestion. Here I was in extreme pain, with a diagnosis of bulging discs, and I was to see a doctor practising hypnosis? I did not voice opposition as I was told that this was a unanimous decision; both my surgeon and personal physician wished me to see this doctor as soon as possible. The secretary gave me the date of my first appointment, which had already been arranged.

As I prepared for this meeting I was both excited by the possibility that I might find some relief and questioning how hypnosis would help me in the short or long term.

Chapter 6

PAIN HYPNOSIS

At our initial meeting, Dr. Hunter reviewed the information on my case that had been sent to her. She told me the reports were concise and accurate based on the condition she saw me in and that they vividly described the pain I was feeling.

She explained the hypnosis procedure and said that with self-hypnosis I might be able to better control pain levels. She said that I would always be in an awakened state and would know what I was doing. (I could not help but think I was always, at least during the day, in an awakened state and knew what I was doing!) The type of hypnosis she was practising did not involve a deep hypnotic trance but one that she felt might help me deal with my problem. She offered to see me weekly for four weeks, at which time she would assess my progress. I agreed to the sessions. There was nothing I would not agree to if I thought it might help.

For each session I sat in a lowboy chair and made myself as comfortable as possible, though it was not easy to get comfortable while wearing a hard collar around my neck. When I had relaxed as much as I could under the circumstances, I would close my eyes as the doctor counted down from ten. Then she would ask me to let my mind wander to some of my favourite exotic places, taking my mind off the pain.

The major problem I had with this procedure was that the excruciating pain I was experiencing was greater than any exotic place I could send my mind to, even though Sasha and I had travelled extensively over the years and I could picture many exotic places. During one of my sessions I told the doctor that for my exotic destination that day I was stepping out on my patio and relaxing at poolside, looking down at the harbour and the city below us. The setting was spectacular, I did not need anything more exotic, but the excruciating, vise-gripping pain overrode the most pleasant of thoughts. It was impossible to concentrate.

The power of positive thinking is strong, but so is the power of debilitating pain. It is overwhelming, especially when it is not intermittent pain but is with you from sun up to sun down as well as through the night. I don't know if someone who has never undergone excruciating skull pain with every head movement could ever relate to what I went through. It could be that only those who have felt such pain can truly understand, which would make it difficult for people who are trying to help.

Dr. Hunter admitted that the form of hypnosis she was using was not a cure for a problem that required corrective surgery, but she said it could help carry me through difficult times. At our last session I asked her for any observations she could make. She noted that I was obviously enduring and tolerating a lot of pain. She also commented that she felt I had become an angry person from such prolonged suffering.

This doctor was not aware of my difficult encounter with the neurologist who had been a discredit to his profession, but she certainly hit the nail on the head with her observation. How else could I feel but angry when a member of the medical profession tosses my head around like a football and leaves black and blue welts on my back? I certainly had reason to question and be angry at such a strange neurological examination. When one was enduring such pain as I was, you do not need to have compounded pain inflicted upon you.

I was overwhelmed with pain. It was my life no matter where I turned or what I tried to do. As much as I wanted to be well, there was nothing I could do. I was struggling with a force so great that it had complete control of me and kept beating me down, even as I continued to fight and cope as best I could from within. For a prolonged period I had been suffering from what I refer to as true pain. In the medical profession it is called chronic pain, which means it has been with you for some time. I have learned that pain can be a difficult problem for the medical profession. At one point I was told I had imaginary pain. I could not accept such an observation as I knew from within my body that there was something seriously wrong. I believe that anyone who is in pain, who sincerely believes there is something physically wrong, must continue to work with a medical team to get to the root of the problem. Even if the pain turns out to be imaginary, at least you will have isolated the problem and can get about resolving it. The main point is to get to the heart of the problem as soon as possible and fix it if it can be fixed. We all know that there is a light at the other end of the tunnel; the challenge is to find the right tunnel.

In this case, hypnosis was a dead end. I was pleased that I had taken the sessions with Dr. Hunter, even though I learned that my positive thought processes, no matter how strong, had no control over the pain I felt. I had always followed the old adage of "mind over matter," and from the hypnosis sessions I learned that I had been successfully practicing self-hypnosis for years, albeit for other reasons than pain relief. All my life I have been a positive person. For years I have been a strong believer in self-talk, accentuating the positive and not leaving room for the negatives to creep in, but now I found that all the self-help self-talk, as positive as it was, did little when I was dealing with profound pain. I had even been using imagery and positive memories to take my mind off my pain for the past few years, letting my mind wander in as relaxed a state as possible. As I was always going to bed in extreme pain, I was usually practising this type of meditation until I fell asleep.

Though fighting and coping with pain was not easy, that was what I must do. I could relax, meditate, dream, and get busy with other things even while the force of pain was with me continually and was powerful, overbearing. I had enough problems without letting negative thoughts creep in, and being positive about my problems by believing they would be resolved helped me keep my mental balance.

The self-hypnosis sessions reinforced what I had already been doing. In my years of working, helping people deal with problems, I had become aware of the dangers of dwelling on negatives. Negative self-talk would make a problem appear worse than it was. People would not sleep at night, worrying about their problems until they became monsters. When I encountered one of these people at work, I would start looking for the positives and firmly entrench them in the individual's mind. Even if this didn't override the problem, it would at least make the insurmountable surmountable. Now I was having to apply this positive thinking to my own problem and it is my firm belief that it played a major role in holding me together through this difficult period.

The medication maze

Early in life I developed a philosophy that there is nothing like nature's own way of healing. I grew up when there were many old-fashioned natural remedies. In the good old days a hot mustard plaster was a common remedy to get rid of a chest cold. If you had a really bad cold you would put a poultice layered with goose grease on your chest. It may sound farfetched, but we used this remedy on our six children and it worked. Whenever we got low on goose grease, we would have a goose for dinner and replenish the supply for fighting the common cold. In those days, even a doctor would recommend a shot of brandy in a given situation. As I recall, it was a topic of conversation when one had to take a prescription drug. Nowadays it seems it is a topic of conversation if you are not taking a prescription drug of one type or another.

Through my life I followed the philosophy that if a pill was not going to help my pain, why take it? I was never one to be reliant on drugs, but in hindsight I see that somewhere, somehow my philosophy went out the window, and over my prolonged period of disability I consumed thousands of pills. No one expected them to heal me; the best they would do was offer some relief. I was hooked on drugs while pharmaceutical companies were profiting. I use the terminology consciously, as the drugs helped me to get by on a day-to-day basis, surviving, existing while I searched for a cure. For the longest time I was like a zombie. How can a human body be mobile and yet so drugged that all it is doing is existing in pain from sun up to sun down? There has to be a better way. I cannot understand how I allowed this to happen, but it is easy to get swallowed up by the system in the hope of a breakthrough.

Over my many years of difficulty I was always disgusted when I was seated in front of my personal physician seeking help and he would excuse himself to his mini-pharmacy of drug company samples. Upon returning to the office he would say, "Let's give this a try." I felt like a guinea pig and I never did get help from these samples.

We always refer to a medical practitioner as "practicing medicine," but when you are down and out you do not want to be practiced on. You want nothing but the cold, hard facts and the proper medication.

If these pharmaceutical companies profess to have so many researched and proven products and if the patient needs attending to now, the doctor should write a prescription and get that patient some relief. In my opinion it would even have been better if my personal physician had been forthright and said, "I'm sorry, we do not have the medication to do the job."

My experience was that I was prescribed drugs on a "Let's see how this works" basis and then kept on the drug for months on end. If there were a sense of urgency in identifying the problem and fixing it, there would be much less stress and less use of unnecessary drugs. There should be a time frame within which a drug is expected to show some positive results. If it does not work in that time, its use should be discontinued. Where a drug is doing its intended job I have nothing but praise for it, but even then, depending on the problem being treated, there should be a time limit for its use. (Perhaps pharmaceutical companies should be required to offer a guarantee and pay a refund on prescription drugs if they cannot do the job intended.)

When the drug you are taking does not treat your problem, you could regress to the extent that a secondary problem develops. In my case, the excruciating pain played such havoc with me that it raised my blood pressure and I had to be treated for hypertension. This was a double whammy from a single problem, as I was consuming even more medication and suffering additional stress. The aim should be to fix the problem and not allow a body to degenerate till it is on the verge of collapsing.

Another negative aspect to these medications is the adverse effects they can have on the patient. A label will state "Could be hazardous while driving." How many patients continue to drive while taking such a drug? And where does liability begin and end if a patient is involved in a motor vehicle accident while under the influence of a prescription drug? If you are taking a drug that can affect your driving ability in any way, should you be forbidden to drive at all? Moreover, what effect does such a drug have on you at work? I know that when I continued to work while under the influence of drugs, I was not performing to my peak capability. In some cases, such drugs could potentially cause injuries in the workplace. Should the label read "Could be hazardous while driving and at the workplace"? Could it be that too many patients are going to work under the influence? That the drug is intended to keep you mobile and going to work even if it is potentially hazardous to others?

As well, the prescription may state that the drug could cause certain side effects and if you notice them you should report them to your doctor immediately. So you report them to your doctor, who decides something does not agree with you and it will be necessary to change the prescription. And on it goes to the next round and another change of prescriptions. One particular drug I was taking required that I undergo blood tests on a regular basis to make sure the drug was not injuring my organs. This testing made me think about how the drugs we are taking have not been tested for our life expectancies, so damage may show up many years after we have used a particular drug.

I believe that when a drug is prescribed there should be full disclosure by the doctor and the manufacturer. What can be expected from the prescription and how soon? What are the drug's side effects? Is it compatible with other medication you are taking? Your pharmacist can provide you with detailed information from the pharmaceutical company or you can go to a bookstore and buy consumer books that list the reasons for taking a given drug and its possible side effects, but I think the patient has the right to know this and should not have to ask for the information or do research on his or her own time. The information should come from the doctor with the prescription and should be written for the layperson as well as the medical profession, bearing in mind that when a patient is taking drugs, he or she may not be able to grasp technical information as easily as usual. It is good to see that in many places monitoring systems are being installed in pharmacies to make it possible to check the compatibility of drugs prescribed to one individual by more than one doctor. There should be a computer file available to everyone attending to you that lists the medication you are taking. This would ensure you do not find yourself in a dangerous situation.

I have actually been blessed with prescriptions that produced the intended results. What a difference this made. Even these medicines may have caused side effects and unknown harm, but at least I gained some relief.

While I give my physicians every credit for doing their best in my case, I strongly feel that drugs should only be used for a set time before a new approach is tried. Intervention procedures should be carried out within a given time frame before undue suffering occurs. I believe that too often the true issue is skirted and temporary solutions tried while the patient's body is subjected to medications it does not need.

My bottom line is, if you are not well and require medication and it helps you, by all means use it. If you are not well and require medication and it is of no help, get rid of it as it is a double-edged sword. First, it is not helping you with your problem. Second, it will no doubt have some side effects. Do not be afraid to be forthright with your doctor about your dissatisfaction with the medication. Remember, it is your body that is being affected. Ask questions about alternative drugs. With so many pharmaceutical companies around, you deserve the best and can demand it. And if there is no medicinal help available, you may as well know it up front and do without.

Finally, don't forget non-drug alternatives. I wrote about health food stores in the Introduction. I had my first experience with these stores when I was being subjected to various forms of medication that literally tore my stomach apart. It seemed that a few of my prescriptions did not have the warning "This medication may cause stomach upset," even though they should have. It got so that I could not keep any food in my stomach, yet I needed what little relief I could get from the medication.

After tolerating this for a long time, I finally pleaded with my personal physician to give me something to settle my stomach. He started to write a prescription, then suddenly tore it up saying, "You will only have to pay a pharmacist for something you can do yourself." He advised me to go to the health food store and buy some Acidophilus bifidus, start taking it right away, and see what happened.

Within a short time my stomach became stabilized and Acidophilus bifidus turned out to be a lifesaver. It restores the correct stomach metabolism required for normal body function. I have used it for over a decade and have not had an upset stomach since. (There is a companion product called Cal'dophilus for people who are allergic to milk.)

There I was in my mid-fifties and this was my first exposure to a health food store. I vividly recall how the shelves stacked with bottled and packaged product had the feeling of a drug store. However, as I looked around I noticed there were also counters of fruits and vegetables, organically and non-organically grown.

I learned that the proprietors of these health food stores are knowledgeable about the various products that they sell and are conversant with the vitamins and minerals required by our bodies, which may be lacking in our diet. I am much more aware of the basic needs of my body as a result of my visits to health food stores. I began taking vitamins to supplement my Commitment to Health diet. Although I cannot definitely prove that they helped me, it is for certain that they have not harmed me. For many years I have also been taking cod liver oil. Here again I have no proof that it helped me, but I do not think it harmed me.

As I am of a Ukrainian background, one of the common ingredients in my mother's kitchen was garlic. Ukrainians love garlic and I can recall how there was always garlic in the soups, the vegetables, and in the roasts my mother would cook. The vegetable salad would have the taste of garlic, or fresh baked bread would be topped with a garlic spread.

Garlic is known around the world for its powers, and scientists are now researching its medicinal qualities and effects on stomach cancer, other cancers, heart disease, and infections. Science and scientists always need to pinpoint the whys and wherefores of a product, but it is a fact that where garlic is part of a regular diet for people in various areas of the world, they tend to be healthier. These people are not concerned about how garlic works. They simply use it as a daily staple.

On that first visit to the health food store I noticed that there was a shelf featuring garlic capsules. I was instantly attracted to the fact that there was garlic advertised and packaged under a number of different labels including no-odour garlic. No clerk needed to convince me that it might be good for me. I bought some and used it in this form for about a year. Then I learned from someone that if you eat some parsley after eating raw garlic in your salad, the parsley will quench the odour. As I was not convinced that I was receiving all the value of garlic from the capsule form, I decided to eat raw garlic every day – crushing it up and then downing it with a glass of water. At first I chewed on some parsley, but I soon gave that up. I see this as taking a non-prescription drug and I can definitely state that the garlic has been significant to my well being. In one way or another it played a part in my overall ability to cope with my crippling pain better than if I had been without it. As well, during those crippling years my immune system was very weak, so weak that I should have been susceptible to the flu or the common cold. Since I started taking garlic I have never had a cold, and I was certainly exposed to cold germs many times.

My experience with walking has led me to view it as the most underrated medication in the universe. It may seem strange to refer to walking as a drug, but I can attest to the fact that if walking has become a part of your life, it is like a drug that must be taken. It gets so that your body craves it, not only on a regular disciplined basis but also throughout the day to get rid of the cobwebs.

Where it may take hours or days to see results from a drug, walking gives instant satisfaction. It arouses every part of the body and it seems like you are gaining energy rather than expending it. Do not be concerned about doing a speed walk or a marathon walk as you embark on this non-prescription drug. Just do it! Even at a slower pace you can cover a lot of ground in an hour. Enjoy the walk, enjoy your surroundings, enjoy the season. Don't underestimate the power of walking.

Chapter 7

THE TRIANGLE

In the fall of 1988 I was on a triangular treadmill with three medical practitioners tracking my destiny. Dr. B, Dr. McNeill, and Dr. Keyes (to whom my personal physician had referred me for an opinion) were all coming up with their observations and suggested courses of action to improve my health. Walking on a treadmill between medical consultants can be frustrating, perhaps even treacherous, like walking on thin ice. You have to be careful and watch for the cracks so you do not go under.

My surgeon had exposed me to a variety of treatments, none of which were helpful but were, in fact, regressive. At this point he was giving me two options: either take six months from work and see if things settled down or have surgery and, all going well, be back to work in three to four months. I discussed these options at length with Dr. McNeill and decided that, in the final analysis, I did not have any choice but to elect for surgery. He agreed, as the MRI had shown definitively that only surgery would correct the problem.

I had seen the neurologist and he had given my surgeon a verbal report. Now I was to see him again so he could discuss his findings with me. Dr. Keyes reviewed the reasons for the tingling and numbness in my hands, but this was not what I had come for. I wanted to know his opinion about the pain in my neck radiating to my skull.

In the course of the appointment I informed the neurologist that I had elected to have surgery and fix the root of the problem. I was amazed at his response. He gave me every reason under the sun why I should at the very least delay surgery, if not forego it entirely. He agreed with my surgeon's alternative recommendation of a six-month rest period, saying I should enroll in and attend a pain clinic. We had a long discussion of this but, frankly, I could not understand how a pain clinic would help if I needed corrective surgery. I had read about and practised so many forms of rest and relaxation techniques that I doubted I could learn more about pain management. I had been living with and managing pain for years and yes, it was a real pain. My recent exposure to self-hypnosis had reinforced my belief in my own pain-management techniques. I was coping as well as I could and it was a debilitating, exhausting, full-time job, one that I could not quit. I had come to the conclusion that I was beyond further band-aid solutions.

The neurologist made a strong case that if I had surgery, I would never know whether the pain clinic would have worked. My rebuttal was that I had been suffering for four years and I questioned how at this late stage a pain clinic could come up with something that would suddenly give me relief. The neurologist told me that the relief, if I were to get it, would come from my ability to better manage my pain. He went on to caution me about the surgery and suggested I get definitive statistics on the success of this type of surgery from Dr. McNeill.

In retrospect I can understand and appreciate that Dr. Keyes made the recommendation he did based on his concern that I could be paralyzed by surgery. This risk was a strong consideration, as was the concern that I might undergo surgery only to discover the procedure was unnecessary. I understand that my doctors had to explore all avenues of cause and treatment for a problem, but after my experience I believe it is important first to eliminate any possible physical causes of pain that might require surgery. There were too many times when my doctors wondered if I was suffering imaginary pain or if I was mentally unbalanced. This in spite of the fact that I had X-rays and MRI results showing definite disc and nerve damage in my spine.

During my lengthy interview with the neurologist I finally asked him if he had ever been subjected to pain, real pain. He replied that he had not, but he was most sympathetic to my problem and knew what I was going through. Asking such a question was not characteristic of me. I don't tend to challenge people whose training and knowledge I respect, but I was at the end of my tether. I wanted to escape this pain if it were at all possible and was prepared to take a risk to do so.

I do believe that the medical person who has never suffered pain is genuinely interested in providing help to patients in pain. On the other hand, I cannot help wondering how another person can know what you are going through when you are the one enduring the pain – it is such an individual experience.

The neurologist had thrown me for a loop. What was worse, in my triangle of doctors only one, my surgeon, had reached a conclusive decision, reinforced by the MRI findings. For a time before my first surgery, Dr. McNeill had felt I should have a triple fusion. We had decided to do one fusion, which may or may not have been the way to go, but now we knew we had a further problem requiring repair.

I did not understand why I could not get repaired if repairing was the answer. I have been a person of action all my life and as a layperson and the one who was doing the suffering, I could see the light at the other end of the tunnel: fix the problem. I could not help thinking of the occasion when my personal physician suggested I see a psychiatrist. I knew I did not need a psychiatrist any more than I needed additional information on managing pain. I knew that there was something drastically wrong with me. When you are overwrought with excruciating pain each and every day for a prolonged period of time, do you need a psychiatrist and pain clinic or invasive surgery?

My next visit was with my personal physician. He had asked me to come in after I saw the neurologist. Here I suddenly found myself in a total turnaround. Up until now Dr. B had been looking to Dr. Keyes for an opinion. Now he was saying I had already had the good care the neurologist was suggesting and I had already benefited from any help I would receive by enrolling in a new program at a pain clinic. Another round of pain clinics would only delay the inevitable. "I think you should have the surgery," he stated.

These were exactly my sentiments and we had a majority in my critical triangle of professionals. Ironic, is it not, that it is finally the patient who must decide what to do? I had faced obstacles along the way, but I was not one to be uncooperative with my medical advisors. I was pleased to know that two out of three – plus the layperson patient, which made it three out of four – were agreed on surgery. Could that many minds be wrong?

At this stage, and because of the many delays and conflicts, I decided I would do a review on paper, setting out where I had been, where I was, and where I was heading. This detailed review helped me reconfirm my decision that there was something drastically wrong with me, that I was getting nowhere in my health recovery, and that I needed to have surgery unless I wanted to be in a collar for the rest of my life, experiencing undue suffering.

The review showed me that I was barely getting through each day. I was eating medication as if it were part of my diet and suffering the after-effects of too much medication. I knew that I was a patient person, but I was beginning to wonder how technologically advanced we actually were. This was the 1980s and I was using all my energy to exist from day to day. I was a disaster trying to hold myself together. I was sick, I needed help, and I was satisfied that the help I needed was further corrective surgery.

I had great faith and belief in my medical advisors, but when all they could tell me over a prolonged period of time was "Hang in there," I started to question what it was I was hanging in there for. I began to fear that I was just hanging in until my body could no longer withstand the stress, until I suffered a stroke and it was game over. With the blood pressure readings I was registering, how much more could my body take? The high stress levels were certainly taking a lot out of me.

I made a commitment for elective surgery to have the obvious problem fixed. The only thing standing between me and surgery was the wait for a hospital bed.

In the meantime I continued going to work every day, even if only for two or three hours. I was getting out of bed in spite of excruciating pain, spurring myself on with positive self-talk even though I was beat before I started work. It was hard to let go and I seemed to get some satisfaction from putting in an appearance at the office, doing some work, communicating with my staff, and going home, maybe with some phone calls to follow up. It was a routine and a distraction from staying at home and suffering. My assistant manager looked after most of the day-to-day business and there was an office manager and three staff people to look after everything else, so I was not needed to keep things going.

Once back home I was walking two or three hours a day even though I felt compounded pain at every footstep. It was a trade-off – my aerobic walking and Commitment to Health for additional pain. There was no escape from pain, but the walking helped me pass the time and keep mind over matter. I got to know many people in our neighbourhood that I would never have met if I had not become ill. It was not uncommon to have someone say hello and add, "I have seen you going by here in a collar for months. What happened?" This would lead to conversation, which also helped to eat up the time.

On the morning of December 15, 1988, however, I was in greater pain than usual when I arrived at the office. I knew I had no business going to the office that morning. I was in such rough shape that I actually hesitated and almost stayed home, then talked myself into going. It is strange, on reflection, how devoted one can be to a workplace, putting career first, health second. I was the only person driving me on.

Once at the office my better judgment told me to forget it, go home. Then I thought, "No, I will phone my surgeon and inform him of my difficulties." But I wondered what good that would do since the pain was nothing new. I considered driving myself to emergency, but discarded this idea as it had never been a solution in the past. I finally decided I would go home, but not until I communicated with my surgeon in another fashion. I felt this would be my last communication with him until I was operated on. I would send a telegram that expressed my faith in him and my reliance on the pending surgery to successfully treat the root of my problem. I wrote:

"The continuing burning, searing, vise-gripping increasing A.M. to P.M. pain continues to test my now marginal tolerance levels daily. I am putting all my faith in you and the pending surgery, which, when I have recovered, will be to me nothing short of a miracle. This may seem like a strange way to further communicate for help, however I believe I have exhausted all of my options."

I was desperate. Obviously I did not expect a call from Dr. McNeill – I was on a waiting list for surgery and had been for some time – and I was fading fast so headed for home.

Four days later, on the morning of Sunday December 18, 1988, I had regressed even more. My whole body was aching and shaking. It was not hard for Sasha to see that I was very sick and she suggested that she take me to emergency at the hospital.

I rejected the offer and said I would make a list of what I was feeling, then phone my surgeon. I was concerned about being bothersome on a Sunday, even though I was in dire straits. My list read:

• *Burning, searing pain in neck area with vise-griping pain into the skull,*
• *shoulders very sore,*
• *compounded tingling in the hands,*
• *severe lower back pain extending to the tail bone right into the crotch area (new),*
• *extremely weak (new),*
• *my colouring deathly (new),*
• *tingling in the toes (new),*
• *loss of balance (new),*
• *the feeling of passing out (new) (all of these old and now new symptoms in the last few days),*
• *there is pain in the jaw (new),*
• *face is twitching (new), and*
• *I am having unusual amounts of saliva.*

After making my notes I had no doubt that I needed to call Dr. McNeill. The hospital receptionist confirmed that he was on duty, but her greatest concern was whether this was an emergency. I did not need to look at the list of problems before me to assure her that yes, it was an emergency.

My surgeon returned my call at around one p.m. and asked me what was up. I told him I was in rough shape. Before I had a chance to review my list he told me to come to emergency so he could have a look at me. My wife must have been anticipating that we would be going. No sooner had I got off the phone than she was ready to leave. She is a careful driver, but on that day I know she wasted no time in getting to her destination.

The doctor treadmill

If you are in pain caused by a problem that requires surgical intervention, have it attended to. Pain is pain, but when it comes from a problem requiring repair, as was my case, four years of torture is too much.

It seems to me we are fighting a paper war, with boxes and boxes of files on a patient when all the patient wants is to get better. Why could a patient not be hospitalized or cared for as an out-patient and be subjected to every test possible *now*, not spread out over a number of years with consultants fighting amongst themselves about their conclusions? I have often heard of patients who are unsatisfied or are unable to communicate with a doctor and seek other help – a referral to a specialist or a second opinion, necessitating more waiting for doctor appointments, more tests.

My advice is to stop, look, and listen as if you were at an intersection or a traffic light. Park yourself as long as necessary and hear what the doctor has to say. Do not be rushed. The worst thing you can do is leave the doctor's office without having all your questions answered. As I suggested earlier, prepare a list of questions that you want answered. Anticipate what you may want to discuss. Do not be afraid you have too much on your list. By the time you see the doctor the question may not be so significant, but you should still search for an answer to anything and everything on your mind. Do not try to avoid any issues. It is extremely important to make a complete disclosure of your problems, otherwise how can you expect to get qualified help? A doctor is not a mind reader and many doctors do not have the probing skills that would be of service to them and to you in getting you to open up. It is important to remember that an incident or symptom that we may feel is insignificant could in the overall scheme of things be important to proper medical treatment.

I believe that if you are having health problems and require medical help, you should make absolutely certain that the diagnosis of the problem and the prescribed medication are to your satisfaction. You must have faith in your doctor. He or she should be able to give you an understanding of your problem and, if need be, a referral for further medical consultation.

If you must get on a treadmill of specialists, inquire about who you are being referred to and what medical specialty they practise. If you have a long wait to see the specialist, ask why. Your problem is not going to get any better while you are on a long waiting list; in fact, there could be some regression in the meantime.

I wonder if it would help to have a medical team, with the personal physician, the specialist, the patient, and a support person who can explain in layperson's terms what the doctors are considering? Too often drugs are prescribed and specialists are called in and the patient has no idea what they are supposed to do. The patient may be able to give the personal physician a response that would show there is no need for the prescription or the referral, but the doctor does not have the time or the probing skills to ask the patient the right questions. A support person could take more time with the patient and gather more details about his or her condition.

If I am sounding tough, I have a right to say it the way I see it as I had to live through horrific, long-term pain – and thankfully have lived long enough to tell my story. In my case, I never doubted my medical team, nor did I ask for a referral to another doctor for a second opinion. When one of my doctors referred me to another, I was willing to try anything that was suggested. The one time I was not willing was when Drs. B and McNeill thought I might need psychiatric help. I felt there was an enormous difference between a deteriorating disc and the imagined pain they thought I might be suffering. I will admit the pain I was enduring was enough to send me over the edge, but somehow I was able to maintain a strained but healthy mental balance.

If you are on a treadmill of doctors, be careful. Are they a result of referrals from one to another at their request, or is it that you have been dissatisfied and continually seek new referrals? I could not see myself going from professional to professional just because I was not getting better. Instead, I saw that there was something wrong and hoped, logically, that it could be fixed. Personally, I always felt positively about the professionals treating me. Yes, there were times when certain comments were made that may have added to my stress, but I did my best to take them in the spirit in which they were given.

On the other hand, pay attention to the source of comments. I do not know how a medical professional can examine you in relation to an insurance claim, spend little time with you, and then literally write a book on your health condition. I do not think these examiners should have access to your file so they can criticize the medical care you are receiving from your own doctor; let them write their own observations. I found these specialists' negative verbal and written comments were damaging and stressful when they contradicted the diagnosis and advice of my own doctors. I tried to take these in my stride, but they did add to the turmoil I was already going through. I had a number of strange examinations and recommendations, all of which ultimately were of discredit to the medical profession and all of which came from the insurance company's medical examiners. Had I followed their advice I could have suffered serious repercussions. Fortunately I did not act without consulting my own medical team.

I never imagined that the problem could not be resolved, though an element of anxiety set in when things were not progressing favourably and I started to question my doctors. We have every right to doubt, just as I found out that the medical profession sometimes doubts our complaints of pain or ill health. I have spoken to many people who had medical problems and many have related how they were told, "It is all in your mind." To a certain degree it is good that the medical profession expresses a doubt; after all, we would not want them to be treating us for something we do not have. However, we want to be treated for the problem we do have and as expeditiously as possible.

Chapter 8

TWELVE DAYS

As is usual at emergency, the routine admissions procedure had to take place, then Sasha and I were ushered to the waiting area. The nurse who was attending to me must have observed my condition and she said I would only have to wait a few minutes. I could not believe how full the waiting room was, even for a Sunday. Obviously we could settle in for a long wait, not a short one.

I was startled when my name was called a few moments later and there was a nurse with a wheelchair. My first thought was, "I did not ask for a wheelchair." It soon became crystal clear that the admitting nurse had wasted no time in treating me like a true emergency.

The second nurse wheeled me to an emergency nursing station and asked me to lie down. She also said my surgeon was already on his way to see me. Within moments Dr. McNeill arrived, took one look at me, and said to my wife, "He doesn't look well, does he?"

We briefly discussed my condition and list of symptoms, my wife related her observations, and his next comment was, "You are staying here." I asked him why I was having so many new symptoms and he replied that when a person had the problems I had, at this stage all kinds of weird things show up.

I didn't see my surgeon again until Tuesday, but other hospital staff gave me a lot of attention that Sunday afternoon, especially after they checked my blood pressure and found it elevated. I was assured this elevation was due to the stress I was suffering, and they had been given instructions on what must be done to make me as comfortable as possible. I stayed in the emergency area until eight p.m., at which time I was taken to a ward and seen by the head nurse on duty.

The head nurse said that my surgeon had ordered I be put in traction to provide me with some relief. For months I had been implementing a form of traction by stuffing washcloths under my chin and around the inside of the collar to take the pressure of my head off the collar. However, in the last while even this was no longer helping me.

By ten p.m., after various visits from staff, I learned they could not properly fit me for traction but that they would do so first thing in the morning. Early the next morning the head nurse came to tell me they were getting things together and would have me in traction shortly. The staff was almost in a panic as they could not locate the necessary equipment and they were concerned about the reaction from my surgeon if they didn't carry out his instructions. As the head nurse said, "We have found we're not prepared for a situation of this type. Somewhere we do have what is needed in the hospital, but at this time we do not know where it is."

It was midmorning when the head nurse came in at a brisk pace and said, "By the way, are you aware that you are slated for surgery tomorrow? We're going to forget about the traction and make you as comfortable as possible for today."

I was frightened and yet relieved to know that if indeed my problem was the 5/6 and 6/7 levels, I could shortly be on the road to recovery. I wondered why my surgeon had not come to discuss this with me, but then I realized that I was no longer a patient waiting for a hospital bed; I was a patient in an emergency situation. I had walked till I dropped.

When my wife came to see me shortly after this she was moved to tears when I told her I was booked for surgery the next day. We both had a good cry and comforted each other. Like me, Sasha felt both stress and a great sense of relief, as she had been going through a traumatic period as a caregiver. In the average home, the caregiver role is not one for which we prepare, and when it becomes a prolonged role it can sap the health of the strongest individual.

That afternoon I had a visit from an anaesthetist. She told me that my surgery would take place the next afternoon at one-thirty. She discussed my general health and said I would probably need some help during surgery. Besides "putting me under," it was her job to monitor my breathing, heart rate, and blood pressure during surgery, to administer the anaesthetic and any other drugs, and to continue monitoring me after surgery till I was breathing on my own again.

Tuesday morning was difficult as I prepared for surgery. I shaved and showered and an attendant shaved my hip in the area where bone would be removed for the cervical fusions. My wife came in early. There was a lot of commotion and the morning seemed to go on forever.

There were more tense moments when I was wheeled away from my room. This was a repeat performance of my first operation a year and a half before. Sasha and I felt all the trepidation and anxieties that accompany major surgery, with the added worry that my health had deteriorated considerably since the 1987 operation. Mentally I was handling the situation as well as I could, but since the previous surgery I had been through the wringer with stress and strain.

The first surgery had been a traumatic and unforgettable experience; this second time felt almost anti-climactic, yet it could not be treated lightly. I knew the potential downside, which was scary enough, and this time I would be having two fusions done, not just one. I could not help but wonder if this doubled the risk of my becoming a quadri- or paraplegic. This possibility weighed heavily on both of us. Sasha had raised the subject on a number of occasions, asking what we would do if I ended up in a wheelchair. I could not bring myself to carry on a conversation about how we would manage if I were crippled. All I could visualize was being myself again and I always reassured her by saying we must see me having successful surgery, recovering, and then getting on with our lives.

Compared to my first cervical fusion, when I had serious doubts about the procedure right up to the time I was wheeled into the operating room, this time I had no reservations. As there was no other medical opinion about why I was suffering such devastating health problems, deterioration at the cervical 5/6 and 6/7 levels had to be the cause. After seeing a variety of practitioners and seeking many opinions, after being questioned about whether my problem was real or imagined, it was me who had to make the decision and I decided to go for the second surgery. I knew I could not go on the way I was and was mentally prepared to lay my life on the line. Needless to say I had faith in my surgeon. My faith kept me going and so did the hope that I would get fixed up and live again, as opposed to trying to exist, which is what I had been doing for a long period of time.

And somehow, deep down, I was always more concerned about my wife than I was for myself. Finally the time came and Sasha and I parted with a warm kiss and clasp of hands that would give us the strength we needed over the next few hours.

The bed ride through the corridors on the way to the operating room was itself stressful. Then I was parked outside a nursing station and visited by different nurses a number of times. Questions, questions, questions. In view of where I was headed I realized the seriousness of the situation and how prepared the operating station must be for me. This was the end of the line and I was totally reliant on those who would be attending me. They say the Mounties always get their man; there is no question that the nurses always get you when you are in a surgery lineup.

As my bed was positioned in the operating room, my surgeon and personal physician came by to say hello. Dr. B wished me well. It was the first time I'd seen Dr. McNeill since I'd been admitted on Sunday. They were the only familiar sights in a room best described as stark and cold. It's scary, but when you are seeking help there is also a comforting feeling that you will soon leave in good repair.

To my right a nurse was preparing surgical instruments; to my left my surgeon was explaining to my personal physician what he was going to do as he reviewed my X-ray charts. It was a repeat of the first surgery and I was again in a state of high anxiety – no doubt this was visible, as various nurses consoled me.

There was some delay in the scheduled start as the anaesthetist was late arriving. In those few minutes it seemed everyone had nothing to do except chat, and I felt so alone.

After the anaesthetist arrived I do not remember anything until I woke up in the recovery room where a nurse was standing over me, working hard to subdue me. I was apparently waving my hands as she assured me that surgery was over and all was well. I vaguely remember being wheeled back to my room and waking again to find my wife at my bedside.

Although I was very sick I assured her I was able to move my hands and feet. This was good news for both of us. We did not talk much as I had heavy eyelids and a sore throat, but Sasha stayed at my bedside and gave me a smile or nod as I was coming out of the anaesthetic. As soon as I could grasp the meaning of her words, she told me that my personal physician had called and told her the surgery went well and the operation was successful. This gave me instant peace of mind. I was all wired and tubed up, a sorry-looking mess, but it was so good to have the surgery over with and I was so pleased that Sasha was at my bedside and had been informed that all went well. It was what we had been praying for.

One could say it never rains but it pours. It was nearly Christmas, though I was not caught up in the spirit of things. One daughter and three sons had arrived to visit for the holiday season and as our daughter and my wife were coming to see me the morning after surgery, our daughter missed the last step coming out of our home, fell, and sprained her ankle. Unbeknownst to me she was in the hospital that morning, getting a cast.

Early the morning after surgery, Dr. McNeill dropped in. He smiled as he approached my bedside, clasped my shoulder with his left hand, and said, "You took a big chance having this surgery. The 5/6 level was marginally healthy but the 6/7 level was so bad there was no disc. It was bone on bone." He assured me the surgery was successful and praised me for being so forthright and honest about my condition, telling me how gratifying it was to find that I truly needed the surgery. One thing I have learned through this ordeal is that one of the biggest problems the medical profession faces is differentiating pain that has an identified organic cause from pain for which no organic cause can be found.

I was able to close a chapter of my illness with dignity as the surgery confirmed what I had felt on the inside: my pain was indeed caused by something I could not handle, a force so powerful it dominated me. I knew there was something wrong and all I wanted was to have it fixed.

Dr. B dropped in soon after this and he repeated that the surgery had been successful. He also emphasized that it was probably the worst case he had ever seen and paid a high compliment to the surgeon, saying what a fine job he had done.

Now I had to regain enough of my strength and get back on my feet so I could go home. Besides the healing that had to take place in my spine, there were unexpected aches and pains to overcome. One of the greatest irritations was in my throat. During surgery a tube was inserted into my throat to carry oxygen and anaesthetic, and as a result I could not swallow anything for the first four days. I was being fed intravenously, so one would think I had nothing to swallow – we don't realize that we continually swallow our own saliva. I was not aware until I underwent this surgery how often and how much moisture is created in our mouths. With my sore throat I could no longer deal with this at a subconscious level. Every time I swallowed involuntarily it was brought to the front of my consciousness. For the next four days I went through boxes of facial tissue, mopping up the saliva. I had no choice.

Before the surgery I had been taking a great deal of anti-pain medication orally. Now painkillers were administered by a needle so I didn't need to swallow the pills. I am not one for needles, but I soon found out that the delay in getting a pain shot was a much bigger price to pay than getting the shot. I marvelled at how I could be in so much pain between needles and yet be relatively comfortable as soon as I had an injection. Needles, needles, needles. As if it were not enough to get them for painkillers, I had quite a round of blood taking as I was running a fever for a number of days. Soon every part of my body was tender from previous shots.

The stitches in my hip also caused a lot of discomfort. The left side of my hip was bandaged with gauze that covered a contusion twelve inches long and five inches wide, narrowing to two inches wide lower on my leg. This was the area where bone was taken from my hip for the cervical fusions. Though the wound was uncomfortable, it reminded me of another risky aspect of the operation that had gone well. The ultimate success of the surgery depended on the proper healing and the acceptance of the bone taken from the hip for the fusion. I later met a man whose fusion did not take and whose surgery had to be performed again. It made me appreciate my surgeon even more and reminded me that when we have health, we must not take it for granted but must make every effort to nourish our bodies properly to maintain that health.

My second day after surgery started out no different than the first. Early in the morning my surgeon dropped by and his visit was again reassuring. He reemphasized that I had taken a big chance, yet the surgery was the only solution to my problem and he was pleased that all went well.

I was struck by the number of people who told me what a chance I had taken. Strange as it may seem, gambling is not in my make-up. However, I do know that I have a "Do it now" attitude if something needs doing. There is a saying "If it's not broken, don't fix it." This always sounded regressive to me, for why would one want to fix something if it was not broken? On the other hand, if it needs fixing, my approach is to fix it now and get on with life.

Dr. B also dropped in and was particularly pleased that my blood pressure had fallen into the normal range since surgery. This was a good sign as I had been taking medication for elevated blood pressure since the cervical collar had come off in September 1987. It is hard to comprehend how devastating the deteriorated disk was to my cardiovascular system. Even though I should have been completely bedridden throughout my pre-surgery period, I had maintained my aerobic walking program. By doing this I believe I unknowingly prepared my body for major surgery. I imagine my surgeon would have been wary about performing surgery had I still been fifty pounds overweight or if my blood pressure had been any higher than it was. I firmly believe my Commitment to Health program had saved my life.

This was another difficult day with lots of pain in my hip and my throat and from the needles. On this day I also looked in a mirror and saw the scar on my throat where the incision was made to do the cervical fusions. It is mind-boggling to think that the surgeon performs the surgery from the front of the throat area, working his way to the inside of the vertebrae to complete the fusion. If anyone ever doubted the skills an orthopaedic surgeon must have, this type of operation would quell the doubts.

The scar from the second surgery was considerably longer than the first. Dr. McNeill later told me this was because the second operation involved two levels of my spine. It seemed odd there was no pain in the area of the incision, but the throat and stitches made up for it.

My dear wife at my bedside these past few days had been a constant comfort to me. Although we did not talk that much, her presence was a form of healing. At times I scribbled notes to her as it was so difficult, if not impossible at times, to talk. She was catching up

91

on her knitting project and socializing with the nurses whenever they had a moment to spare. I have nothing but high praise for the way the nursing staff took care of me, as I am certain they do in all hospital environments. They are a dedicated group of people, proud of their work.

Friday, December 23, I was visited by a colleague of my personal physician. Dr. B was to be away for the next five days and this fellow was keeping an eye on his patients. I'd met him a few years earlier when he was filling in for Dr. B at his clinic. At that time he asked me how I had managed to lose so much weight. I described my Commitment to Health program and his response was, "I will have to try that." What an endorsement. Today he observed that I was doing pretty well in view of the type of surgery I had come through.

For the first time since surgery I took a few swallows of my breakfast, lunch, and dinner, though I felt guilty about sending most of the meals back. This was part of the road to recovery. Each swallow was slow, accompanied by great burning pain, but after that day I knew the next one would be better.

Later that day a physiotherapist dropped by to fit me with a new Philadelphia collar. I was told I would be wearing the collar for the next three months, twenty-four hours a day, in and out of bed.

Every day after surgery is a big one in one way or another. The fourth day presented another hurdle to overcome as I was told that I had not had a bowel movement for four days. Very casually the nurse added that they would give me something mild to churn things up.

I had woken up with an appetite and though I still had to force-feed myself, seeming to take forever, I cleaned up the tray. I was congratulated as the tray was taken away, and good news travelled fast as virtually every nurse that morning commented on the fact that I had eaten my breakfast. My doctors were pleased with my progress, the nurses were glad to see me eating and starting to talk, the physiotherapist had me out of bed for a few minutes, and I found out how weak I was.

My stomach kept me awake a good part of the night with a lot of false alarms. In the morning on the fifth day after surgery, however, I rang the nurse for real, was assisted to the washroom (my first walk since surgery), and was back to normal with my bowel. This proved to be the first of a number of visits to the washroom and they totally played me out. How quickly we weaken when bedridden.

I continued to have my share of painkillers, but I could see that I was getting better, albeit slowly. The well-wishes from family, friends, and colleagues were coming in the form of cards and flowers, and my room was looking as festive as it did after the first surgery. I was often brought to tears at the outpouring of friendship.

As usual, Sasha spent the better part of the day with me, but this was to be a first in our married life. We had been so engrossed with my hospitalization that we had barely noticed the holiday season was upon us. For the first time in thirty-seven years we were spending Christmas Eve together in a hospital. Our quiet time together was most meaningful as we had so much to be grateful for.

Christmas day in a hospital was certainly not in my plans for December 25, 1988, but the way my health had been in recent months I did not have the strength to make too many plans about where I might be on a given day. Certainly the medical profession had been occupying a lot of my time, as I was theirs.

On awakening on Christmas morning I gave special thanks to the good Lord for the greatest gift of life and for the successful surgery. Even though I was still feeling weak and sore, I managed to wish each of the nursing staff a Merry Christmas. My window sill was a living Christmas tree, decorated with a variety of colourful plants.

Christmas dinner at twelve noon was a full-course turkey dinner with all of the trimmings – a tribute to the cook and staff who prepared it, for nothing had been left out. I was most impressed but also saddened by the fact I was having Christmas dinner alone without family for the first time in my life. Nevertheless, I was not alone as it was never quiet during the day in the hospital.

In the early afternoon I knew my wife was on her way while she was still quite far from my room in the hallway. I could pick out the sound of her footsteps even if there were a number of people walking down the hall. This day a special warmth ran through me as I heard her footsteps. After all, it was Christmas day.

Sasha's Christmas wishes were heartwarming, and for the first time in many months I could see some of the tension leaving her. It had been a long, hard struggle for both of us, and throughout it she had been a support for me. Our marital and love relationship had grown strong over the years, we were virtually inseparable, and we both cherished it, yet the recent difficult times put a great strain on our marriage.

My wife, a woman of many talents, designs a greeting card for our friends each year. For this Christmas she had done a pen-and-ink Christmas rose and all of the nurses on staff received one of her cards. They were most appreciative of this special thought and it provoked a lot of comment. Many came in to request her autograph on the card.

This was the fifth day after surgery and I soon found out how weak I was. I got out of bed, went to the washroom on my own, and with the help of a walker, slowly maneuvered out of the room, past the nursing station, and back. I was completely exhausted, but it felt good. I had been for a short walk and once I got back in bed, that was it for the rest of the day. Sasha was both pleased and displeased with my venture, but I needed to test myself and push myself if I was to get better.

Sasha and I had a lovely visit in the afternoon and then she went on to spend the rest of the day with family. For our Christmas evening meal in hospital would you believe they gave us each a hamburger? And did it ever taste good. It was obvious I was starting to feel better, as I cleaned up all my meals on Christmas day. After dinner I thought I would go for another short walk, but I could not muster up the strength do so. I had exerted myself enough earlier in the day.

December 26, Boxing Day, my surgeon dropped by and was pleased with my progress. Although sympathetic to my desire to get back on my feet, he reminded me that I had gone through serious surgery only a few days earlier. Before he left he told me that he would be off for the next week, but depending on my progress and how I felt, I would be able to go home towards the end of the week. That was good news. Although I appreciated the hospital care, there is no place like home if you are able to manage there.

At this point I was still on intravenous and taking antibiotics for a fever. I ate all my meals on this day, used the washroom on my own, and again made my way past the nursing station to the end of the hall, crossed over to the other side, and worked my way back. My second day out of bed, albeit not for long, gave strong indications that I was on my way. Sasha was concerned that I was overexerting myself. Whether I had overexerted or not, I again found that this was my only walk for the day. There is an old saying "By the inch it's a cinch," and I kept reminding myself it was a blessing that I was already up and moving about.

By the time the physician arrived on Tuesday, I had shaved, cleaned up, eaten breakfast, and with the help of a cane, which was my newest means of support, had already been for a walk around the hall. The use of the cane was necessary because I was very weak. It also allowed me to favour the hip area where the stitches were.

This day was my best yet. By evening I had made three rounds of the hall and was feeling quite good, though I needed all the rest I could get in between each walk as the effort totally exhausted me. My Commitment to Health program was already urging me on.

Wednesday, Day 8, I reported to the associate physician that I was not resting all that well, my blood pressure at rest was 120/70, and my shoulders and back were quite sore, but otherwise I was taking my meals and everything else seemed to be working well. He reminded me of the major surgery I had been through and added that I was up and about quite a bit and the use of a cane could give me shoulder pain. Strange trade-offs, but I figured that if I was going to get better I had to keep testing myself and my progress. Before Sasha left that afternoon I told her that if all was well the next day I would probably elect to go home. This didn't entirely meet with her approval as she could see how weak I still was, but she was also happy to see that I was feeling ready to leave.

By the time the associate physician came in on Thursday, I had already advised the head nurse I wished to be discharged. The physician agreed there was no place like home and was pleased to see me feeling well enough to go home. He stressed that I was more than welcome to stay longer if I needed to. I told him I was still not resting well and that I hoped the quiet of home would be helpful.

The nurse on duty packed my belongings for me and about eleven a.m. the ambulance attendants were there to pick me up for the journey home. The staff expressed their warm wishes, and I could not thank them enough for their help. Then I was on my way. The ambulance ride home was comfortable. I was lying down and my neck was not subjected to the stop and start motions as it would have been had I been sitting up.

There was some maneuvering around our pool and patio to get me to the front door, and I reminded the attendants I did not wish to go overboard. They assured me they would get me inside safely. Once in the front door, all I could do was make it to the nearest chair. They were on their way and I continued on to the comfort of my own bed. It was great to be home and no longer in the pain I was in when Sasha took me to the hospital twelve days earlier. It was hard to believe how much I had gone through in such a short period of time. Although the trip home did not take that long, the excitement and preparation before I left the hospital and the excitement of getting home did me in for the rest of the day.

Stress, distress, and how to handle them

I have provided detailed coverage of these twelve days in hospital to show the stresses and benefits that surround any type of surgery and to emphasize how we must remain positive in any given situation. It is often difficult to do so, but, barring physical complications, I believe our attitude has a lot to do with the recovery process. In my case, I felt a miracle had been performed in view of the progression from excruciating pain to relative comfort.

The lesson I drew from the events described in this chapter was: if you have something wrong with you and it can be repaired, don't put yourself through pain and suffering by delaying surgery. I went through sheer agony for sixteen months and all it took was twelve days in hospital to put me on the road to recovery. If only medical science could have seen from the outside what was going on inside, I would have been spared prolonged pain and various types of manipulation that proved to be regressive and stressful. Stress causes distress and distress will cause a host of problems that get so intermingled they can make it impossible for the medical profession to identify where the root problem is.

Stress is part of life and probably has been as long as humans have inhabited the earth. However, we have our own peculiar stress factors to deal with as we move into the twenty-first century. With our high-tech communications we know of world events literally moments after they have happened. The news media, the bearers of good and bad news, have the stresses of the world before us on a minute by minute basis. Some people start taking this news personally and get so that they cannot take any more of the global stress.

But narrowing our focus to our immediate surroundings does not eliminate stress. Look at the stress a child faces growing up today. When he or she is a teenager, the pressure builds even more. Children try to grow up too fast, live in fear of the high expectations their parents, teachers, and society have of them, and too often turn to alcohol, drugs, and violence. Everyone is getting stressed out.

Adults confront many stresses in the daily routine. These regular stresses are a way of life and most of us learn to cope with them in a regular manner, though we receive no lessons in being an adult. Unfortunately, other people find coping with these stresses too difficult and seek band-aid solutions. Alcohol and drugs provide an escape for many, often ending in death. Our society tries to cope with and help these people, but it is becoming increasingly difficult as the disease of stress spreads. It is self-inflicted and this is what is so hard for the user to overcome.

Then there is the stress of the post-retirement period. After enjoying a relatively healthy life, the aged all too often start to deteriorate rapidly. It is sad, in a way, as they have worked a lifetime and provided for retirement only to find that they may not enjoy the fruits of their labours.

An important thing to keep in mind is that we are here on this earth for a relatively short visit. We are only passing through and sometimes we must recognize that a stressor is outside our control and not let ourselves get caught up in it.

However, this is not to say we should ignore all our problems. There is another aspect to stress that many people do not understand and, therefore, do not deal with. When we ignore stress or pretend that it will go away, it can become compounded stress, an even bigger problem. The key is to deal with it as quickly as possible – isolate it, alleviate it, or at least get it under control.

Most people are aware when they are feeling stressed out. This awareness is probably even stronger when they are alone, with no one to confide in. In cases like this, we are not aware of the fact that we are our own worst enemies. Let me explain this comment, drawing on my own experiences. Over the years I have met individuals who were down and out, fully stressed, in distress, with a multitude of problems. When I did some soul-searching with these people and asked them how they spent their day, how many people they saw, who they talked to and about what, and then narrowed it down to hours, I often found that the troubled person did not spend much time out of a twenty-four hour period talking to others. And even if he or she did spend a fair amount of time with others, how many hours of the twenty-four did they still have to themselves?

My point is that in a twenty-four hour day, of all the people we have contact with, who do we talk to the most? To be certain – ourselves. And who do we listen to the most? Again, it is ourselves. Self-talk is a natural mental process. What goes in also comes out. The more positive thoughts we dwell on, the stronger we are. The more negative thoughts we dwell on, the weaker we become.

It is obvious that the person who is in a stressful position, whether the stress is caused by school, job, finances, health, marriage, or anything else, is in trouble and needs help. The stress is severe and may be compounded the more they talk to themselves about it. If they are repeatedly talking garbage to themselves – i.e., blaming themselves for the problem, insisting to themselves that there is no solution – that garbage will pile up so they end by having a garbage dump in their own mind. Think of a landfill. Eventually it becomes full, is capped, and could be turned into a park. But that doesn't change the fact that it is all garbage underneath.

In the case of our thought processes, it is imperative that we learn how to get rid of the garbage in our mind and replace it with good thoughts before our mind is filled and destroyed. It can be done, but one has to work hard at it and, most of all, believe in oneself. We must be able to deal with the garbage in – garbage out thought processes quickly or they will destroy us.

In the months and years following my neck injury, I learned what stress was.

• Stress is when, in that split second of the accident, you are overcome with fear.

• Stress is when you are coping with pain and it is interfering with your work.

• Stress is when you are seeing your doctor and he apologizes for the fact that he cannot help you.

• Stress is when you are in physiotherapy and the treatment is causing your health to regress.

•Stress is when your family sees your condition and knows there is nothing they can do. This is double stress, for you and for them.

• Stress is an insurance adjuster who tells you there is nothing wrong with you.

• Stress is an allergic reaction to the iodine dye used in a myelogram.

• Stress is being told that you have to have surgery that could cause you to become a quadri- or paraplegic.

• Stress is surgery.

• Stress is finding that your blood pressure is elevated to life-threatening levels.

• Stress is having your doctor tell you he does not think you are crazy but that he wants you to see a psychiatrist.

• Stress is recognizing the stress that your caregiver, your wife, is being subjected to.

• Stress is coping with contradictory medical opinions.

• Stress is losing touch with business colleagues and friends because you are ill.

• Stress is losing your job or business enterprise, or giving up a life-long career.

• Stress is living with the unknown for years on end.

• Stress is not being able to do the things in life that are important to you.

Many of the stressors were with me for the duration – the pain in my neck and skull, for example, and the worry about how the stress was affecting my wife and family – while others popped up from time to time or caused a great deal of stress for a short time – like the worry about coming out of a surgery a quadri- or paraplegic. In many instances there was absolutely nothing I could do except muster the strength and perseverance to continue to cope with the problem. What I attempted to do with these stressors – I believe successfully – was take each of them and replace it with a positive, an alternative. I tried to sort them out and get rid of them as quickly as I could. The mind has a great recall of negatives and it can be difficult to block them out, but when I put them to paper I could review them and exorcise them rather than allowing them to build up in my mind.

I would make a list of problems and worries. On a second sheet of paper I would divide the stresses into two columns labelled "I Can Do" and "I Cannot Do." Rather than having all of them cluttering my mind, they were now cluttering the paper and I dealt with them as I could. I had to be strong within myself, believing that I could deal with these problems or, alternatively, making myself stop worrying about the ones that were outside my field of influence. My attitude to my problems ultimately determined my attitude to recovery – and this attitude was transmitted to all the people who were dealing with me.

I discovered that stress can lead to distress, so it was important that I tried my best to cope with the situation, keep an open mind, and play it cool, rationalizing every move. ("Play it cool" refers to the ability to assess what has been said, by whom, and how much it contradicts other professional opinions, and then evaluate how useful it is.) Finally, it was important to recognize and trust my gut feelings when it came to evaluating my condition and my ability to deal with it.

Stress is controllable, but it must be handled in a mature, forthright, expeditious manner, preferably in such a way that you can get rid of as much of it as possible every day. If you can't eliminate it, you must learn how to cope with it or, ultimately, be able to recognize when you cannot handle it on your own and seek professional help.

If you are currently barraged with problems, no matter how few or how many, get out a pen and notepad and start jotting them down. This exercise can be surprisingly therapeutic. Just identifying problems on a notepad will give you a sense of control. Take the time to categorize them in terms of priority and identify those that you can immediately work on and take care of on your own. Having done this, you are already on your way to getting rid of some stress. Other problems may take longer to deal with, but at least you have identified them and are working on eliminating them. You have lessened the stress load. If there are problems for which you need professional help, the fewer other stresses you have to deal with, the stronger you will be to deal with those difficult stressors.

Again, the aim is to get rid of stress as quickly as possible and to gain control of stress that cannot be immediately eliminated. Trust yourself and your feelings. Don't let others tell you that you do not feel what you know you feel. Don't let them blame you and don't blame yourself for things that go wrong in your life. Take responsibility, make apologies if need be, but don't let failures and mistakes eat away at you. Don't forget the power of positive self-talk.

Chapter 9

ABILITY VERSUS DISABILITY

Once I was home from the hospital, I knew I had a lot of work to do. Getting well is a full-time job if you are determined to do everything possible to expedite your recovery. You are on your own now, no longer subjected to medical care twenty-four hours a day, and it can be a lonely road. In my case, I was always reaching for something to do within my limitations.

On my tenth day after surgery, my first day at home, I felt very weak. I had more than my share of pain and I was bedridden and disabled. Personally, I did not and do not like the word disabled. It is too harsh, but it was a reality I had to face up to.

Rather than have breakfast in bed, with the help of the cane I made my way to the kitchen table. As I left the bedroom I walked the length of the hallway, then came back through the dining and living rooms to the kitchen. I walked slowly, very slowly, and I found that my mind was working overtime. As I made that horseshoe through the rooms I counted thirty-five paces. With approximately three feet to the pace, those thirty-five paces meant I had just walked 105 feet. On my first day home I made that walk five times. I had walked about a tenth of a mile.

I could have felt sorry for myself – it was winter after all, cold outside, and the easy way would have been to stay in bed – but instead I was already back to my Commitment to Health walking program. I found that since I had walked on a daily, disciplined basis for such a prolonged period of time, it had become ingrained. It was a habit and a necessary part of my daily routine. The desire to walk was so strong that it was fulfilling when I did it. It was like the need to drink water daily. I cannot stress enough: if you are reading this book and have not taken up walking on a daily basis, do it now. It is one of the least strenuous aerobic exercises, but it is good for you and will add years to your life.

By the fifth day at home I was walking half a mile. They say that we walk great distances every day without realizing it, whether it's at home or in the workplace. I believed it now that I had estimated the distance I was walking in the house. It gave me a great sense of accomplishment to know that in spite in my condition I was walking a good distance, albeit slowly and carefully.

As it was winter I had wondered how I would start to get mobile, but here I was right in my own home with the solution. The days passed and I was soon walking a mile a day and doing it in under an hour. A mile an hour is a snail's pace, but I made myself feel better by telling myself that at least I was moving about. For every negative thought I created a positive one.

After two weeks at home I ventured outdoors on a nice day with my wife at my side. To our neighbours I appeared to be a cripple, using a cane, wearing a cervical collar, and making every step a careful one. It took fifteen minutes to walk to the end of our crescent and back. Along with the walk, the fresh mountain air did me in and I returned home to rest and read.

For the first few weeks my wife insisted on accompanying me when I went outdoors. I was grateful for this, as one never knows what could happen. It also meant that she was getting outdoors and getting some exercise, even though the pace was slow. Because I was favouring my hip where the stitches were pulling, my body would twist with each step. On more than one occasion my wife burst out laughing. When I asked her what was so funny she replied, "You walk as if you had crapped your pants!" Whether that was true or not, I was now able to relate to many people I had seen walking with a cane, doing a shuffle, walking with difficulty or very carefully. I came to understand that they moved that way because they were favouring a certain area of their body.

Within forty days of surgery I had built up from a fifteen-minute walk to an hour each day. I walked at a steady pace with no stopping, and my wife began to notice the effect this exercise was having on her thighs. I guarantee they were not getting bigger.

In spite of my ongoing discomforts I knew that I must continue my exercise and walking program or I would seize up. As it was winter and rainy, I knew it would be the easiest thing in the world to talk myself out of a walk on a rainy day. Instead I took the opposite approach. My Commitment to Health was foremost, rain or shine, I would dress warmly and take my umbrella – and yes, you can stay relatively dry with a big umbrella. Going for a walk in all weathers accomplished two things that were important to me. I got fresh air into my lungs and I got the exercise that was both good for me and had a tiring effect. I would rest after the walk and it would be a better rest than I had without the fresh air and exercise.

As I rested, from our bedroom window I could look out to our backyard where we had a bird feeder. With fresh snow on the ground it was a picturesque sight. I always had my binoculars at the bedside and watched the constant activity. I discovered that bird-watching is most fascinating and I could spend hours of enjoyment in this tranquil, quiet setting.

I also spent much time reading. The week before my surgery I had stopped at a bookstore to buy a copy of *Eat to Win*, by Dr. Robert Haas, for a friend who was to have open heart surgery. (Over the years I had recommended the book to a number of my friends.) When I was in the bookstore I also picked up a book called *Controlling Cholesterol*, by Dr. Kenneth Cooper. It was Dr. Cooper who I had heard speak on the aerobics of walking at one of our conventions, and I felt his book should be good reading. This book was my bed partner when I returned home from surgery. It was my first major introduction to the subject of cholesterol. I read the book while I lay flat on my back, a few pages a day. I could not help thinking that the average person should be more informed in this critical area. It is important to know what is good for us to eat, what is bad for us, and what we can do to improve our general health. If we become knowledgeable soon enough, we may implement changes and perhaps live a longer, healthier, more fulfilling life.

In the book, Dr. Cooper refers to cycling as an excellent aerobic exercise. Cycling had been a major activity in my life up until my accident. Sasha, our children, and I all had bicycles, though I had never used cycling as a daily aerobic exercise. This is the difference between activity on occasion and a daily routine. I would cycle, but it didn't help my weight or my health because I didn't use it daily in a disciplined manner.

Now, however, with my fusion on the mend and my health improving, I asked my surgeon if a stationary bicycle could help my recovery. He endorsed this type of activity as long as I was properly fitted with my cervical collar when cycling.

One of our sons was visiting from out of town at the time. He checked out the market for me and brought home a shiny new stationary bicycle. I was like a kid with a new toy, though careful not to overdo it.

Getting the stationary bicycle brought back memories of my wife's uncle. Over thirty years earlier he had suffered a stroke and was much incapacitated. At that time, stationary bicycles were just starting to come on the scene and they were expensive. Sasha and I were in our early years of marriage, starting out on a tight budget. Since her uncle lived in our area, I wanted to get him a stationary bicycle so he could exercise, but I could not afford to go out and buy a new one. I decided to improvise instead and went out to buy a used bicycle, then took it to a welding shop where they built a solid frame for the bike to sit in. My wife's uncle was elated when I brought the bicycle into his home. What made it worthwhile was that he used it each and every day. He could slowly turn the pedals while fighting a crippling disability. Again I emphasize that we must discover what we can do for ourselves to help us on the road to recovery.

In March 1989, three months after surgery, Dr. McNeill told me to start removing the collar for up to two hours a day. I did not have to take it off for two hours straight; instead I could break it up into ten- or fifteen-minute blocks so long as they added up to two hours a day. As it turned out, I was not able to remove the collar for a long period of time without a lot of pain setting in. This was difficult to accept as since the surgery I no longer suffered the excruciating pain I had felt before surgery. Moreover, I was no longer stuffing the collar for additional support. Nevertheless, I carried out the instruction faithfully.

On my next visit, in early May, I saw a locum instead of my surgeon who had gone on leave himself due to a disability. The locum was a fully qualified orthopaedic surgeon and I was comfortable with him. I told him I had a lot of neck pain and discomfort radiating to the skull. The locum said that I had worn a collar for such a prolonged period of time that my neck muscles had atrophied. The pain was caused by my starting to use these muscles again. It could be quite a while before I was out of pain, but I must continue to increase the time I went without the collar, building up to eight hours a day. He added that I might have to learn to live with a certain amount of permanent disability, but if I were not successful in getting by without a collar, I would be in it for the rest of my life.

Here I had been looking forward to getting better and going back to work, but now I faced a new set of circumstances. I was in a "Damned if you do and damned if you don't" position. I would gain relief from extreme pain if I kept the collar on, but the longer I wore the collar the longer it would take to get past the pain. I had the mental ability to get back to work, but the disability was like a noose around my neck - or in this case, like a cervical collar.

The doctor said I should try to get back to as many of my normal activities as possible, including swimming. A bear for punishment, I complied and started to keep the collar off for longer periods of time with no relief whatsoever. I had the philosophy of "No pain, no gain."

We were having some wonderful spring weather that year. On Mother's Day the sun was shining and it was like the middle of summer. Our pool was a warm 80 degrees Fahrenheit and I decided that I would go for a swim. I did about six laps of the pool and then stopped for a rest. When I got out of the pool I wondered what was happening to me. My hands were tingling more than ever, there was nearly unbearable pain in my neck, and I was shaking as I had never shaken before. My first reaction was to wonder what had come over me. I soon realized that I was not ready for such exertion.

I made another visit to the locum and he decided to enroll me in a water physiotherapy program at Lions Gate Hospital. He said I should stand in the water up to my neck and let the buoyancy of the water hold my head up. This would allow my neck muscles to rebuild, but it would not cause as much pain because I would not have to hold my head up against the pull of gravity.

I began attending these group sessions. As I stood in the water, the physiotherapist, who was also in the water, led us through a series of exercises. I found that I was not only limited as to the number of repetitions I could do, but I also could not keep going for the full session. This was the first exposure I had to others who were working to build muscle tone in various parts of their bodies. I noticed that these other people would yelp when they were testing their body beyond its capability. I continued the program for some time and also did home sessions as we had a swimming pool, but there was no noticeable progress. I went to the Thorson Rehabilitation Clinic, a fifteen-minute walk from our house, for biofeedback sessions and cortisone injections into my neck area. And all the while I continued my walking as that, along with my exercises (see "Use it or lose it" at the end of this chapter) and daily water therapy, was about all I could do.

The locum had told me it would be a slow process. I was beginning to wonder what the word "slow" meant when it came to healing and rebuilding muscles. It was one thing to recover from a potentially crippling disaster - my car accident and the subsequent disc deterioration - yet here I was with another form of crippling that left me in absolute pain as I entered the recovery process. I was blessed to have come through two serious surgeries that took care of my problem. Unfortunately, my prolonged immobilization in the cervical collar produced another problem that I had not expected. I recalled how my doctors had been hesitant to recommend use of the collar. It was the last resort and now I knew why. This reinforced my philosophy of "If it's broken, fix it now." The long delay before surgery had contributed to the wasting of my muscle.

I just had to keep going. By the end of the summer I was still using the collar a few hours a day, but I forced myself to be without it as much as possible as I did not want to have a noose around my neck the rest of my life.

I could drive the car and was managing to get to my medical appointments on my own, though my driving time was restricted. I also started to build model airplanes, a hobby I had enjoyed as a child. It was fun and brought back many fond memories. I built three airplanes and when I let my grandchildren fly them, I soon found myself doing repairs as well.

I was grateful that I was able to do as much as I was doing, that I wasn't so crippled I could not function on my own. At the same time, I *was* a disability statistic. Even though I had the ability to do things, there was always an overriding pain. Yes, I had a limited ability to move my head sideways and up and down, but not without compounded pain radiating into my skull with every movement. It got so that even when the collar was off, if I had to move my head to one side or another I would turn my body from the shoulders up. It became natural to move in this manner to guard myself against pain.

I had been told that I must continue to be patient, that the daily healing process was microscopic, that it could well be a couple of years before I was able to return to work. This was another blow and it was hard to take, but it still left me with a light at the end of the tunnel if I only persevered. I was determined to do so.

Use it or lose it

In my chapter on "Vital Signs" I mused about how we take for granted all of our various body functions. What we tend to forget is how finely tuned all of the parts are and how misuse or overuse or even a minor change can affect their operation. For example, think of the star hockey player who suddenly experiences problems with his knees, the golfer who finds a minor accident affects his swing, the tennis pro who has sprained an ankle and cannot participate in an important tournament.

I could go on with such high-profile scenarios, but it is interesting how the average person also often complains about the loss of full use of body parts due to injury, surgery, inactivity, overactivity, or old age coming on. Many problems result from our need for rest and relaxation, but along with this we need to keep our bodies limbered up. We understand how a professional athlete can run into problems, but we don't realize how many demands we put on our own bodies and how much we take good health and strength for granted. Like the athlete, we've got to keep our body exercised and in shape to meet our needs.

I used the following exercises, adapted from various exercises learned in athletic programs while I was young, to keep myself limber before and after surgeries or when I was confined to bed for long stretches of time. I believe they are part of the reason I was able to start getting around as quickly as I did. Perhaps they even shortened my stay at the hospital. I would urge anyone who does not exercise daily to adopt some or all of them for plain old good health. If you follow this exercise regimen when you are bedridden, you will be exercising vital parts of your body and ensuring better health from doing so. (One proviso: If you are recovering from surgery, ask your doctor what you can or cannot do and remember that it may well be that your own body will dictate your limitations.) If you are in the hospital recuperating from surgery, make sure the nursing staff is aware of your activity or someone could walk in on you and think you are going bonkers.

I suggest that you do your exercises at a regular time, preferably a time when you are unlikely to be disturbed. If you like tranquillity, as I do, it can be a wonderful quiet time. Alternatively, you can turn on some music of your choice.

• Exercise #1 – Lie flat on your back, hands by your sides, take a deep breath slowly and exhale slowly. Repeat a minimum of ten times but build up to as many as you need. For anyone who needs relaxation, this exercise is a must.

• Exercise #2 – With hands by your sides, clench both your fists, hold for five seconds, and release. Do this a minimum of forty times. Build on that number if you wish. This is an excellent exercise for your hands and for relaxation. As you clench your fists you can simultaneously clench your stomach and relax. It will tighten your stomach muscles.

• Exercise #3 – With both hands by your sides, move your wrists back and forth twenty times, then roll both wrists the same number of times.

• Exercise #4 – Lie down with your hands clasped on your chest. Pull your right shoulder and arm upwards. Hold, then release. Do the same with the left shoulder and arm. You will feel the pull of the muscles in arms and shoulders.

• Exercise #5 – Repeat exercise number two, but this time clench your fists and hold for ten seconds. Do a minimum of ten, building up to as many as you want. This is a tension soother and I can recommend it whenever you are feeling bottled up. It can be done in the comfort of your favourite chair at home and even one hand at a time while driving your car.

• Exercise #6 – Pull your stomach muscles in, hold, and release. Repeat ten times. This is different from exercise number two and harder because you do not have the extra support of your clenched fists.

• Exercise #7 – Raise your left leg, bend it, place your foot on the right knee, then return left leg to prone position. Repeat ten times. Reverse legs and repeat the process. Feel the muscles stretch?

• Exercise #8 – Starting prone with your legs outstretched, clasp your left knee with your hands and slowly bend the left leg, bringing it back as far as you can. Hold for thirty seconds. Repeat the process with the right leg and feel the pull on the muscles.

• Exercise #9 – Lying flat, bend your left leg and bring it back as close as possible to the buttock. Hold for ten seconds. Repeat the process with right leg.

• Exercise #10 – Sitting up, clasp your left leg at the knee and pull the leg towards your body. Repeat ten times. Repeat with right leg.

• Exercise #11 – Raise your left leg, extended, five times. Repeat with right leg.

• Exercise #12 – Raise left leg and twist to the left and then to the right five times. Repeat with right leg.

• Exercise #13 – With feet outstretched, move your left ankle in a circular motion forty times. At first you will find this quite tricky, but persevere. Repeat with right ankle, then repeat the process simultaneously with both ankles. Concentrate on making a perfect circle.

• Exercise #14 – With both legs outstretched, let both ankles move in unison back and forth to the left and to the right. Let yourself go, do as many as you can.

By now you have given your body some excellent stretching exercises and also some relaxation. During my recuperation period I did these exercises daily, three times a day, for many months. I did as many repetitions as I could, given my medical condition, building up slowly as my health improved. Along with medication and hypnosis, I believe they were helpful over a prolonged period of time.

When we are bedridden and immobile our body is both at rest and seizing up. By maintaining a minimal exercise program, no matter what your condition, you will be helping your body to keep in shape. If you cannot do all of them, do some of them. Start small and build, but do start. You can even use your imagination and create your own exercise program. I guarantee that it will be helpful.

Chapter 10

MAKING A MOVE

In May, five months after my surgery, I received a phone call that was to be yet another test of my strength. I had been away from my office since December on a short-term disability program, and I had planned to, and been assured by my doctors that I would be able to, return to work within six months. However, I found I was still in rough shape.

On this day, an executive from my employer company called to ask if I would be back to work before the six-month short-term disability period expired. His call came on a very difficult day and in fact I was in bed when the phone rang. He told me that he did not like to be the bearer of bad news, but if I was unable to be back to work within the six-month time frame, the company would have to appoint another manager and I would be on long-term disability. There was no discussion. I knew that I would not be well enough to be back to work and I told him so.

I'd been struggling with my pain. Now, with the ring of the telephone, I had given up my management position. In retrospect, I was shocked at the way this was handled and wondered if all such situations were dealt with the same way. Was there no compassion, no feeling, no thought given to the mental state or physical condition of an employee receiving such a call? Was this the best way to tell an employee that such a decision had been made? More importantly, was it the best way to tell a person in poor health? Bad news is hard to handle at the best of times; when a person receiving it is lying flat on his or her back, such a call can have an unduly negative effect. Granted, I couldn't carry out my duties and I understood the company couldn't hold my position open indefinitely, but surely there was a softer way to communicate such a decision. As it was, it did not compound my pain, but it did leave me totally stressed out. It took a lot of strength to get through that day, and it took some time to get over the shock.

By early fall I got an okay from my doctor to go for short trips in the car. Except for visits to medical people I had not been anywhere since my surgery in December, so it was good to get out. With Sasha driving, we started going for half-hour jaunts, slowly increasing to an hour. We tended to get out on the freeway for these drives so as to avoid the starting and stopping that jerked my neck and increased my pain.

Eight months of confinement is a long time and I did all I could to stop it from dragging me into the ground. I read a lot each day, everything from insurance industry news, periodicals, and books to financial papers and our daily newspaper. There were times when I was scratching for something to read by the end of the day and on one fall day in mid-October that is precisely what happened.

I'd read the newspaper, but I was still hungry for more. By chance I opened the paper to the country homes and acreages section of the classifieds. A small ad for an executive home in the country on an acreage caught my eye. I cut the ad out of the paper and left it on the side of the table until I was going to bed, which was relatively early by any standards. At that time I took the ad to Sasha and asked, "What do you think of this? I thought it might be nice to use it as an excuse for an outing."

She read the ad and replied, "I would love to see the property."

The next day I called the realtor and arranged for us to meet in a designated place from which we could drive to the property together.

The drive out to Chilliwack took about an hour and a half, and by the time we were halfway there I was ready to turn around and go home. I was in a collar during the drive and in progressively more pain, but I did not want to spoil Sasha's day. She had given up a lot of her time for me and I owed her this outing. I would persevere, put mind over matter...but nothing would stop the pain.

We met the realtor at the designated spot, introduced ourselves, and agreed that I would ride with him and my wife would follow us. We travelled the main highway for about four miles and then turned onto a gravel road that seemed to twist and turn forever up a hill through a densely forested area.

For the second time I was ready to turn back, as I was suffering additionally from the twists and turns in the road. I was not feeling at all well, but I did not want to disappoint the realtor as well as my wife.

The realtor finally made a turn into a driveway. The first building we drove by at the gate was a log construction that was literally falling apart. As we drove down the private road I could not help wondering what would be next.

We turned onto the paved driveway and arrived at a home on the hill. Motorists driving by would never know it existed. The realtor showed us the house. Both my wife and I were most impressed with the property, even though our visit was the result of curiosity and, more than anything else, a need to get out of the city where we had been virtual prisoners in our own home for many months. We discussed the price and the property's good points, and then I told him we would want to think about it. Having said that I thought to myself, "What are you talking about? You came out for a drive, not to think about a house. Or is this a polite way to escape from the realtor's clutches?"

The realtor went on his way, as did we. I could tell my wife liked the home, and certainly it exceeded my expectations. When we were about ten miles from the property I said to Sasha, "Let's go back and buy it."

Sasha must have thought I was even sicker than she'd imagined. She quickly gave me reasons why we couldn't buy the house, ending by pointing out that we'd only come out for a drive. Besides, we already had a home in which we had agreed to stay until we could no longer manage on our own. We had long-term plans in place, carefully thought out.

However, we continued talking as we drove home. Sasha admitted that she had fallen in love with the property. She had grown up in the country and early in our marriage we had lived in a rural area, so yes, she could make a change. But she pointed out that I had my career to consider.

I assured her that my career would be with me wherever I might live. I had years of sales experience, sales management experience, and my CLU designation. No one could take that from me and I could set up as an independent insurance agent in my home if I wished. I told her there was another angle we should seriously consider. According to my doctors it would probably be two years before I could return to work. I felt that living in the country on an acreage could be conducive to my long-term rehabilitation.

I knew I would have to do a lot of talking to persuade her as she was not even nibbling, but by now I was in a disastrous state. The outing had been too much for me. I should not have attempted such a trip, but my philosophy was, "How will I know where I'm at unless I test myself?" Test myself I did, on a daily basis. I tested and pushed myself to such an extent that I took walks a number of times a day and for fairly long distances. To my wife it seemed like I had only returned and I was on my way again. I was proving to myself I had the ability to keep fighting the disability.

For the next couple of weeks we discussed at length the property we had seen. Normally if you are out shopping for a new home you do a lot of looking. In our case, we saw one piece of property where the primary purpose was an outing in the country and we were now talking about buying it. At the same time, we were having a new brick enclosure built for the fireplace in the lower level of our North Vancouver home, and we were adding a new bathroom and new carpeting. Our plans were to stay, not move.

But still we considered the possibility. I called my company's head office, told them I was thinking of buying a property out of town, and asked if they'd be agreeable to my opening an agency in this rural area when I was able to return to work. The response was favourable, although it all depended on my health. The realtor called to ask if we were still interested in the property. I told him I wanted to come out again and asked if it would be possible for the owner to be there and to identify the corners of the property as I wanted to know where the boundaries were. Arrangements were made. This time I was not just going out to have a look. If I was satisfied with everything, we would buy the property. Whether we were buying or not, we decided we would stay in the area overnight as the trip both ways on the same day was too much for me.

My wife was both excited and frightened. Here she was with a sick husband on her hands, in the middle of having renovations completed in our home, winter was setting in, and now I had decided to buy her the home in the country that perhaps she had told herself she would never have. But I had resolved that I would not let my health stop me from buying this property if at that crucial moment of decision everything was favourable. Nothing would stop me from starting fresh, and I was in the position of starting over in any event with regards to my work and my health.

We went out to see the property. The realtor and owner showed me the source of water, the property boundaries for the seventeen and a half acres, and the home. It was raining and I was not well, but I was determined to complete my inspection. I asked the agent to write up an offer and told him where we would be staying overnight. By midmorning the next day the agent called to tell us that our offer had been accepted. We would take possession in the spring.

My wife was elated. My first thoughts concerned how we were going to sell our current home in the middle of winter, especially since we were a month away from completing the renovations. It doesn't rain but it pours, and this type of activity is for the healthy and able, not for someone disabled as I was. It is not easy to push onward when you are not well, but I also felt there was an element of rehabilitation attached to this move. I had hope and faith that all would work out and that maybe leaving behind an environment where I had suffered for so long might not be all that bad.

In the midst of this, another bombshell dropped. Dr. B had recently given me a prostate examination and he wanted me to see a urologist. "Heaven help me," I thought. "Here I am in plenty of pain already and now I am to be subjected to painful rectal examinations." I was thoroughly examined, tests were done, and on a second visit the urologist, Dr. Mike Sookochoff, told me I had to have a Reagan operation. I had never heard of such an operation, but the urologist told me that at that time prostate surgery was being referred to as the Reagan operation because U.S. president Ronald Reagan had recently had a prostate operation. (Ironically, our new home was on Nixon Road. I seemed to be moving in presidential company.)

I had my health to look after, the prospect of prostate surgery, the sale of a home, plus a move in the spring – no small task for a healthy person, let alone a weakening zombie. However, I knew I could stand up to the challenge. After all, that had been my life story. If I did not have a challenge on any given day while conducting business, I soon set out to create one. I thrived on it, though I would be the first to admit I was not thriving in my attempt to get better and resolve my neck problem. I was existing with a disability, yet it seemed I could always raise the strength and the ability to face new challenges.

And I took on one more challenge. Over twenty years earlier I had purchased a 1931 Model A pickup truck as a retirement restoration project. This truck sat in our backyard, waiting for the day that it would return to its original shining splendour. I decided that I might as well have someone else work on the restoration since I couldn't do it in my current state. It would be a kind of rehabilitation project for me. I'd be able to drive over and see how it was coming along, health permitting, and it seemed a more rational decision than simply moving the unrestored vehicle with us to our new home. I made arrangements for the restoration while coping with my neck and head pain. As always I was a bear for punishment, yet I continued to take an active interest in life.

Our home went on the market in late December, an experience in itself. We had one of the worst snowfalls on record. My wife got the house ready to show on a number of occasions, only to have the realtor cancel as we were snowed in and the clients could not make it up the mountain drive.

The weather improved by February 1990. One week our realtor told us he would not hold an open house the following weekend as he was going to be in Florida for a convention. I asked if he would mind if we put up the "Open House" signs ourselves and let the public come through, as we would be at home anyway. He agreed, so we prepared to hold our own open house. That weekend the weather turned summerlike. I uncovered our pool. It was crystal clear, inviting enough for a swim. I set out all our patio furniture around the deck as well. It added a positive ambiance, but it was also very much a part of the property for sale.

Early in the afternoon, one woman and her realtor spent a lot of time looking at the property. Before they left they told us they would be returning shortly, as the woman wanted to bring her husband to see the house. It wasn't long until they returned, and their realtor told me that he felt there would be an offer before the day was out. That evening we did receive a call from the realtor who was covering for his

118

colleague in Florida. To make a long story short, the property was sold. There were three other follow-up calls from people who had seen the property that weekend, and all were disappointed when they learned that it was off the market. We arranged for the new owners' possession date to coincide with the date we took possession of our new home. Now we were into the next challenge of preparing for the move.

I took on the task of packing our dining room dishes. It took me a week. I wrapped every item individually, and wherever I set a box for packing, that is where it stayed as I could not move anything of substance. My wife and I packed light, fragile items a few at a time, our children helped when they could, and we were fully prepared for the big move when the day came.

During this period of selling our home, packing, getting ready to move, having the Model A hauled away, and preparing for prostate surgery, I certainly had my share of distraction from my disability. My days were so filled you would think I'd be able to forget the pain. Unfortunately, this was not the case. I fought the pain continually. No matter what I did, there was no relief; whenever I did anything, I would end up being sick. Every movement of my head brought me additional pain and at times I could not help wondering whether I had rocks in my head to be making such a major move when I was so seriously ill.

My response was to carry on, repeating my mantras: "Ability over disability." "Mind over matter." They played a big part in my continuing to fight this extreme neck pain on a daily basis. And throughout all the commotion I continued to take my daily walks and my rest periods, visited the doctor, and arranged to have my prostate surgery in February prior to our move. This was another test of my positive frame of mind over matter and my ability to take charge while suffering from a crippling disability. I could easily have rationalized postponing surgery until I was well. However, I knew that if I did not have my prostate taken care of, it could develop into an explosive situation. (As an aside, I advise all male readers to have annual prostate checkups after the age of forty. Prostate cancer is easy to deal with if it's caught early. Why neglect our bodies and find ourselves dealing with a monster?) I was in Lions Gate Hospital from February 11 to 17, 1990, for the surgery. I was not confined to bed when I returned home, but I moved slowly and carefully for the next couple of months.

From the time we purchased our new property until the day of the move, my wife was out to the house a number of times, either on her own to check the size or aspect of our new rooms, or with family members who were anxious to see what their parents were up to. As for me, I did not visit the house from the day of the purchase until the day of the move. I was too sick to go anywhere except for short outings near home.

We had favourable weather for our moving day at the end of March. It was exciting, frightening, and also somewhat emotional as the realization set in that we were leaving our home of many years. My wife had become skilled at observing when I was in particularly bad shape, and she had already planned how she was going to deal with me on moving day. As we had two cars, it was a foregone conclusion that each of us would drive separately to our new home on the day of the move. First thing in the morning, before the movers arrived, we finished packing the car I would be driving out. I did not know it, but Sasha had decided that I would be leaving within the hour. It did not take much for her to convince me that I would only be in the way. I put Ricky, our red Persian cat, in his cage and we were on our way.

I'll digress here for a moment to tell the story of Ricky, who by this time had been with us for many years. One day I happened to be visiting one of Vancouver's animal pounds on business. When I was leaving, I noticed a sign on the bulletin board that said a home was needed for a red Persian cat. When I asked to see the cat, I was taken to an area of cages where a beautiful fluffy red cat looked me right in the eye. I fell in love with him instantly and asked if I could take him home with me. The nurse was not sure if the cat was ready to leave. She excused herself for a moment and returned a few minutes later with a veterinarian. He opened the cage door and raised the cat's head, looking under his chin in the throat area. I noticed a triangular shaved spot under his chin.

When the vet said the cat was ready to go, I asked about the shaved spot. The vet told me that only a few days earlier, Ricky had saved the life of another cat. Apparently this other cat had been hit by a car. He had undergone an operation, but he needed a blood donation to save his life. Ricky happened to be chosen as the blood donor. Over the years, whenever a visitor remarked on what a stately cat Ricky was, I would tell the story of his blood donation.

Ricky and I arrived safe and sound at our new home. I brought him into the house and had a good rest, as I was totally played out from the drive. By late afternoon the movers arrived and it was interesting to see the swift, orderly manner in which they unloaded the vans. All boxes and furniture were marked with stickers that indicated the rooms they were to be placed in, so the movers were able to drop everything off in its designated spot.

Sasha had anticipated it would be a long day for the movers and had prepared a nice dinner for them. This gave them the energy to continue unpacking and by eight-thirty in the evening the move was completed. All of the major items were in their places, the beds were set up, and we only had to unpack the boxes, which we did at our leisure.

After the movers had left and we were preparing to settle down for the evening, we called Ricky in but he did not respond. We learned the next day that a cat will often get disoriented in new surroundings. By the fifth day when he had not returned, we were very worried about him. I went out to walk down the road and back, calling him. When I returned, my wife called me from the patio to say that Ricky had just come home. We were so pleased to have him back.

It was good to be settling into our new surroundings and in some ways it made the events of the previous six months seem like a dream.

Do not give up

I have described our move in detail because I want to emphasize that even if we are disabled, we all have certain abilities and we must continue to use them. This in itself is a big healer. It would be detrimental to do something physical that is beyond our capability, but there are so many ways in which we may continue to be active. I believe that, above all, we must continue to have an active mind.

Living with a crippling disability – and I use crippling in broad terms – is a full-time job. Rehabilitation is also a full-time job. It is a job for which we have no skills and it requires self-training, self-discipline, mind over matter, strength, and high degrees of faith. You are not interviewed for the job or asked for your qualifications; you suddenly have it, no questions asked. You will not know until you are disabled if you have the ability to cope. A disability will sap your strength at the same time it tests you, demanding strength far beyond what you think you have. The key is to have a positive outlook on both life and the disability you are coping with.

The ability to have faith and belief in yourself and in others (doctors, caregivers, technicians) who will take care of you in your disability requires tremendous strength of mind – even more so when you hear of the negatives related to your condition. It is so easy to give up hope, to stop struggling against pain and disability and sink into depression when you think there is no escape, but in times such as these you must be able to rationalize and seek out the positives.

Do not give up. I know it is easier said than done. When you are seemingly boxed in with nowhere to turn, your medical help at a standstill, why keep fighting? You are given little if any encouragement. You are seeking that ray of sunshine at the other end of the tunnel and there is not so much as a glimmer of light. The roof has caved in and you are lost, quickly losing faith in the high-tech medical system that has no answers for you.

You must not let this happen. There is so much to live for and yet in troubled times one can easily say "For what?" It would be so much easier if you were fighting to a known goal, however this is where the challenge becomes even greater.

My experience dealing with many problems over the years has taught me that there is a sure way to solve problems that takes advantage of our positive and negative self-talk: writing them out. It takes a little more time than mulling things over in your head, but it's worth it. As an example, in my late twenties I was in business for myself. I was giving a lot of thought to a major expansion that would have required many thousands of dollars, a lot of money at that time. The plan was risky and this was bothering me. Even though I already had the cooperation of the bank to finance and proceed with the project, I decided to set the whole scheme out on paper.

When I wrote out the plan with the positives and the negatives, there were a couple of negatives I could not get rid of no matter how hard I tried. They were the same negatives that were churning through self-talk when the plan was not on paper, but they were so much more final in pen and ink. It did not take me long to decide not to proceed with the project, and I could have saved a lot of time, thought, and worry had I put the project on paper in the first place.

Taking a pen and paper and writing out the problem at hand is a means to an end. It may sound strange, but when you write something out, somehow it takes on a different appearance. By writing out the positives and the negatives, it could turn out they are all negatives, and it certainly allows you to see the bigger picture. More importantly, once you have committed your situation to writing, your mind is free to come up with even deeper positive and negative thoughts that you have not yet considered.

Do not attempt to open and close the file on the same day. Remember that, generally speaking, a problem is the culmination of matters over a period of time, and you need time to think about it. The key is to diarize new thoughts or problems as they come up. What will happen is that, with time, you will get the picture in written form. It may be a paragraph, a page, or pages of written material. It matters not how much; what matters is that you have something constructive to work from.

I say "constructive" because I believe that using self-talk alone, and mentally piling up our problems, puts us on the road to self-destruct. It may be that when you see the big picture in writing, you will solve your own problem. On the other hand, you may learn that you require appropriate help. But even if you need help, it will be easier for another person to help with your problem if it is written out clearly.

To confirm that my suggestion is both sound and healthy, I will give a medical example, though you may be able to think up examples from your own life.

When you see a medical practitioner, he or she will take a medical history and record information on areas of your health that do not seem at all relevant to your current problem. This is done so that pertinent data is not only recorded but is on file for future reference. From the big picture that develops, the medical practitioner may find a pattern of material to solve a problem.

In your own case, you may find that as you write out your thoughts and problems, you start seeing a pattern of behaviour or events that explains a problem you are having or answers a question that is bothering you. Again using my case as an example, I found it frustrating to divert all my energy to the problem of pain and healing and still get no results. No matter where I turned, I was no better off. I was not well, literally cut off from the rest of the world, and there was a lot of time for thinking and self-talk. However I refused to give up the fight and found that pen and paper proved to be a part of my salvation. I made notes of my thoughts, my questions, and things that I could do to use my time within my limitations. I had no time for garbage as I had one goal in mind: to get better and get back to work.

It was not easy, and as the months turned into years I had a lot of time to rediscover myself. However, there was nothing to rediscover. Nothing had changed other than the fact that I was faced with a crippling, painful, debilitating disability. There were many times when I was in extreme agony and I would divert my thoughts from the pain by telling myself how lucky I was. How lucky I was that I had all my faculties, could take care of myself, and how, with time, I would get better. Then there were times I used to think that there might be a medical breakthrough. Wishful thinking on my part, but at least it was positive.

I fed myself a lot of positive self-talk on a daily basis, which was sometimes hard to digest under the circumstances. When you tell yourself you are getting better when in fact you are regressing it is not an easy pill to swallow, but I was determined not to give up and to this day I do not know what the alternative would have been. There is no doubt in my mind that had it not been for positive self-talk, I could easily have succumbed to the pressures of pain and frustration that I was subject to. This is the power of determination.

Chapter 11

OUR HOME IN THE COUNTRY

The weather continued to be warm and springlike after our move, and we were able to enjoy the fresh air and the view from our patio from sun up to sun down. Our property sat on a hillside 800 feet above the floor of the Fraser Valley. A good part of it had been cleared and left as pasture. The rest was what I would call firewood bush. Twelve fruit trees adorned the pasture. When we got around to doing some pruning, our neighbours told us the trees had probably not been pruned in over forty years. The land was interestingly contoured, as it was hilly with a gully running along the southern part of the property.

In the gully ran a fast-flowing stream that provided a substantial amount of the drinking water for the town of Chilliwack, which was below us some six miles as the crow flies to the west. This stream ran from the range of mountains behind us – the Cascades. From our kitchen window we could look out to the mountains and a cascading waterfall. From other rooms in the house we had a 360-degree view of either snow-capped mountains – the Coast Mountains and the Cascades – or the beautiful fertile Fraser Valley that was in splendour throughout the year. The Fraser River ran east to west below us, taking on a different appearance summer and winter. It was spectacular. We'd lived on a mountainside in our previous home, with a major city and harbour below us, but this was a fair trade.

The property was part of a homestead originally settled in the early 1900s. The residence, of post-and-beam construction, was situated so that it caught the sun rising in the morning and enjoyed natural light till the sun set in the evening. At the gate stood a structure made of hand-hewn logs, in total disrepair and apparently ready for demolition. My mind was awakened the first time I saw it, and you shall read the results of this later in the chapter.

When we originally looked over this property, I was so sick that when we got home I could not help thinking I was crazy for considering a purchase. At the same time, I was so impressed that I was ready to buy on the first visit.

As I thought about where I stood with my health at the time, I could picture myself healing in either place. However, there was a difference. Rather than being confined to a city lot, I would have an acreage. Rather than walking the city streets, I could walk the country road. Most significantly, I recognized a feeling of serenity, privacy, and peacefulness in the property, and I needed all of this and more during my rehabilitation. I felt that in the long term there would be many pluses in the country property to help me maintain the strong hopes of recovery I had.

It was not a dream come true. It was not as if we were out looking at properties; this was the only one we looked at. It was not that we had planned to make a move. It probably would never have come to pass had I been healthy and working. It was fate and I believe there was a power that led me to read the advertisement that changed the direction of our lives.

As we settled into our new surroundings I continued to have a lot of difficulty with my neck, but I resolved to manage as best I could. I had learned to cope and cope I did, although with much pain. I found a local physician, Ron Bull, to monitor my progress. I recall he just shook his head on my first visit as I did a capsule review of my problems. I saw him every month. At times it must have been nerve-wracking for him to see such a wreck each month, especially given the minuscule progress I was making.

We spent a lot of time outside. The property was nicely landscaped and needed minimal upkeep, but grass keeps growing, especially when you maintain it with proper fertilizing, so there was lawn to mow. When I say "lawn," I am talking about a large area – three quarters of an acre. I decided that I would add a new activity to my daily Commitment to Health program. I would walk behind my self-propelled lawn mower for the necessary five hours of maintenance. I spread it out over two or three days, with lots of rest in between.

I found a large overgrowth of wild blackberries on the hillside. These occupied a nice strip of land, and the more I looked at them the more I wanted to get rid of them. With a set of pruning shears and leather gloves I proceeded to snip these thick vines a foot at a time, making neat little piles of brambles that I later carried to a large pile for burning. I clipped and snipped for an hour or two a day through the whole summer, and I did it on my hands and knees as I could not bend over without excruciating pain. Where there's a will there's a way and if I could, I would find it. When the job was done, I was surprised how much space those blackberries had taken up. I could have hired someone to destroy this growth in a matter of hours, but if I had done that I would not have been able to enjoy the peacefulness and serenity of our field, not to mention the distraction of the hours clipping vines.

Since Sasha wanted a garden, we soon arranged for a local farmer to till some land for her and she was soon happily planting and weeding. I planted some Italian garlic just to see what would happen. I had been eating garlic for years but had never grown it. In fact, I had never planted anything before. We also planted some rhubarb and it was fascinating for me to see it grow.

When the fruit trees bloomed they were a sight to see, especially as they were sadly overgrown. We could not see through them, there were so many branches. We did not harvest much fruit that fall and learned it was because the trees needed pruning. Year by year we had main branches cut back on each tree, and by the fourth year they had taken on the shapes of an artist's dream. The real bonus was that we began to harvest four to five boxes of apples from each tree. We gave many away and stored the rest through the winter. Sasha baked fresh apple pies right into March, when our supply ran out. The trees produced apples of a species that was no longer commercially available. This added to our enjoyment of them.

That first fall we took our garden in and had a supply of vegetables for the winter. I was absolutely elated with the harvest of the garlic – homegrown garlic, grown in soil that had not been tilled for over forty years, and the first thing I had ever grown myself. I had also planted some elephant garlic and was amazed at the result. Elephant garlic is just that – huge, elephantine. The bulbs at maturity will have four or five cloves, sometimes more, but the size of the full-grown garlic is a sight to see. The biggest heads of garlic came in at eight and a half ounces – half a pound. I could not believe something had grown to such a size in our garden.

A couple of rows of garlic does not a farmer make. However, this experience made me think about my previous vocation, at the opposite pole from working the soil and planting seeds, and I considered how wrapped up we get in our own vocations, whatever they may be. My vocation in the life insurance business was a career that occupied as much time as I would give it. I made sure to spend time with my family and to take vacations with them, but when you are operating a business there is only so much time available and it never seems enough.

Now I learned that those who grow garlic are also devoted to their chosen vocation. I discovered that there are garlic conventions and they are major events. I could relate to an insurance convention or other types of professional or industry conventions, but a garlic festival was difficult to comprehend. I don't know why this was so. After all, when I had bought garlic in the past I had not taken it for granted. I should have realized garlic production was a highly specialized agricultural field and there must be a vast organization of growers to put this product on the shelves. But up until this point I had never related to the garlic growers or thought of the great satisfaction they must realize when they harvested such an incredible product (bear in mind that garlic is a non-prescription drug that has been around for centuries and is known for its recognized yet unexplained medicinal properties).

No doubt it is the same with anyone, in whatever vocation, but the point I want to make is about the size of our little worlds. Since moving to the country, in spite of a severe handicap, here I was doing things I had never done before. And although both the type and amount of my activity was still restricted, at the end of the day I had satisfaction knowing that I had accomplished something.

One other activity that first year involved the windowless, two-storey, hand-hewn log cabin at the entrance to our property. We learned after we moved that the log house had been built in 1912 by Henry Nixon, a local settler, who used logs from the property. He had raised seven children in the two-story home, which was twenty by twenty-six feet. Now it was weathered on the outside and was full of junk and wood. I walked out to the cabin every day and slowly started clearing the debris from the building. As I did, I discovered how rotted the joists and floor were. In addition, the staircase leading to the second floor was in bad shape. On closer examination I found that the building had been built on tree stumps. These were rotted out and the building was slowly sinking as the rot progressed. I made arrangements to have a carpenter come out on Saturdays to do some preparatory work and build forms, then we poured a new cement foundation, lowered the building to solid footing, and began to remove and replace the main floor and the staircase and rebuild a twenty-six-foot porch that had originally been part of the building. This project kept me busy and distracted. (Ultimately the restoration took four years. We built a new roof with hand-split shakes from cedar logs felled on our own property. New windows and frames were built by a craftsman who replicated the originals. A third of the main floor was redone with salvaged material from the old floor and the rest covered with salvaged fir flooring from a home demolition in Vancouver. I never tired of the project physically, as most of the work was done by outside help, and as the activity extended over a long time, it kept my interest and attention engaged.)

I was no longer wearing my cervical collar. My neck and head movement was restricted and I could cause myself compounded pain with the wrong type of movement. But I had learned to be as cautious as possible and there were signs of some relief. This was turning out to be a therapeutic healing environment beyond compare.

Winter started in early November with subzero temperatures and gale-force winds. The high winds caused power outages; we were without power at least twelve times that winter. One episode lasted for five days. However, we had our oil furnace as well as an ample supply of firewood for the fireplace to keep us warm. I found the winter went by fairly quickly. I did a lot of reading, went through my files, and did some writing and with visits from family and friends who dropped in, the season slipped by.

At Christmas our family visited and we had, as always, an enjoyable time. By seven-thirty or eight p.m. I would excuse myself for the evening as I could not take the pain without lying down for some relief. Tolerating the literally intolerable on a daily basis over such a prolonged period of time took a tremendous amount of my strength. I discovered I had an inner strength and faith more profound than I could ever have imagined. The will to live and live fully, no matter how much I hurt, kept me going.

One evening when there were high winds and the power had gone out, our family looked over the valley below us and watched a spectacular show as the electrical transformers blew, lighting up the sky one after the other. The waterfall froze over completely, like a large, majestic icicle.

At the end of our first year on the property, as spring was finally breaking, we could not help but wonder if all our winters were going to be so bad, but we learned that winters come in cycles of varying severity and this winter of 1990-91 had been the most severe one in over fifty years.

My daily walks continued and by now I was acquainted with all of our neighbours, not that there were that many. Everyone got to know Duchess by name and someone once referred to her as "the Queen of the hill." It was a good feeling when neighbours stopped their vehicles to exchange pleasantries as they passed on their way up or down the hill. Stopping to say hello to great neighbours is a wonderful way to start a day.

The long hard winter had given me a lot of time to think about what we might do with the hilly but arable land on the property. I decided to start a tree farm, so that spring my sons planted over a thousand trees – a mix of Douglas fir, Grand fir, Scotch pine, and Norway spruce. They did the work while I supervised, and again I found the project to be most therapeutic. Even though I could not participate with the planting, I was doing something tangible and it gave me a good feeling. When you are suffering on a daily basis you can stand a lot of good feelings.

I also planted more elephant garlic – this time a fifty-pound bag I purchased from a grower who specialized in growing commercially and selling seed stock. I now had garlic-growing fever, albeit in a small way, which gave me an interest and something to do.

That spring Sasha had a bigger garden. She planted some strawberries, raspberries, and blueberries. Without question the property was proving agreeable not only to me on my road to recovery, but also to Sasha, who I believe is a born gardener. Her father was a wheat farmer and she grew up on the farm, and one could tell where her roots were.

I mentioned earlier that I had a 1931 Model A Ford pickup truck that I purchased in 1968 with plans to restore it when I retired. When we moved from Vancouver to our country home I had the pickup delivered to a shop for a restoration from the ground up. Although I did not do any work on it, a visit to see the truck became a destination outing for me and helped consume many hours, giving me a distraction to keep me busy during a difficult time. When it was returned to me in like-new condition, I took the pickup to various country parades, local fairs, and even won a first prize in its class at a Concours d'elegance vintage car show. Sasha and I enjoyed these outings and the chance to talk to many people who fondly recalled these old vehicles. The smiles on their faces as they reminisced and had their pictures taken by the truck made me feel good inside. (Over the following years I also bought and had restored a 1953 Pontiac Chieftain two-door hardtop as a fortieth wedding anniversary gift for Sasha, and a 1937 Ford pickup.)

As spring rolled into summer I was feeling better, stronger, with much more neck mobility. I was off pain medication except to handle the occasional flare-up. Dr. Bull was pleased with my progress and did a good job of keeping the reins on me.

Part of this involved my vocation. Everything I did was with an eye to the day when I could get back to work. I had renewed my licence to practise each year during my disability period so I could start up again as soon as I was able. I felt that I was ready to start thinking about going back to work for a few hours a day. I discussed this with Dr. Bull. He was cautious, telling me that though I might be feeling better, I must be better for some time before I went back to work. Based on my past experience, I had the sense to accept his opinion. I did not want to regress, as he suggested I would if I started to push myself too soon.

I continued my rest and relaxation periods, my walking and limited daily activities. In spite of limitations my days were full, and each and every day I had a deep feeling of accomplishment.

Our children visited during the summer, and two of our granddaughters were with us during the month of July. On the day before their departure we decided we would treat the girls to a movie, *101 Dalmatians*, playing in a neighbouring town.

It was a forty-minute trip, so Sasha drove. Then she went shopping while I took the girls to the movie. On our way back to pick up Sasha after the show, a vehicle came out of a side street into a main intersection, right into my lane, and I hit it broadside.

Chapter 12

SPLIT SECOND

It was as if I were in a demolition derby. In that split second a vehicle was in front of me and there was no time to do anything but hit it. If I applied my brakes it was at the point of impact; there had been no time to apply the brakes and skid into the collision.

The vehicle I hit spun around a couple of times and came to rest some distance from the point of impact. Inside our car I had two distressed granddaughters. They were crying, screaming, and very frightened. The older girl bit the inside of her mouth and the other was petrified as she cleaned away the blood from a nosebleed. I was already shaking and experiencing increased pain in my shoulder, neck, and skull as well as in my lower back, extending down my leg to the right foot.

Many things happened quickly – offers of help, witnesses coming forward – before I even had the opportunity to recover from the shock. One woman who had witnessed the accident asked if there was anything she could do, particularly when she looked in the car and saw two frantic young girls. I said I would be grateful if she would drive to the designated spot where we were to pick up Sasha and bring her back. Luckily I remembered what she was wearing and the woman was able to spot her quickly. Before the car had even been moved from the site of the accident, Sasha was back consoling our granddaughters.

By now the police were on the scene and shortly after that the cars were moved away from the flow of traffic. The police took statements and told me that the other driver had been charged for failing to yield.

I had begun to shake immediately after the impact, but now I was shaking hard and uncontrollably. I was in obvious distress. Sasha tried to convince me to go to the hospital's emergency room, but I insisted instead that we get transportation home. There happened to be a car rental outlet at the corner, so we rented a car and headed home. By the time we got there I was in compounded pain. I phoned Dr. Bull and he told me to take an increased dosage of the pain medication I had previously been taking.

By the end of the day our granddaughters had settled down but were still very disturbed. I recalled how, when we left the movie theatre, I checked each of them to ensure they had their seat belts fastened. I dreaded to think what might have happened to any one of us had we not been buckled in. Although my wife and I were uncomfortable about their leaving the next day, after a telephone conversation with their parents we agreed to let them go. They arrived home safe and sound but, we were told, still upset.

Within days I had new pain in my right hip and knee extending to the toes. There was debilitating stiffness in my neck area and I also felt severe pain in both arms, extending from the elbows to the shoulders.

I went for my daily walk and with each step I felt compounded skull pain. Every time I moved my head in any direction I felt compounded pain radiating to the skull. At night I was resting with the soft collar on. I say "resting" because I was not sleeping well at all. This had turned into a new nightmare, as if I had not already suffered enough. I was back to lots of rest, medication, self-hypnosis, hand-clenching exercises, daily sessions in the hot tub, ice packs, hot packs...and nothing was working. I was in total distress and absolutely helpless after years of healing.

When I rode in the car with Sasha driving, I felt additional pain radiating to the skull with every start and stop of the vehicle. It was a repetition of what I had already been through and it was severe, with no let-up whatsoever. I was an absolute wreck. I was also "gun shy," flinching at the sight of any vehicle that showed the slightest inclination to make a wrong move.

My doctor sent me for X-rays, but they showed no visible damage. Dr. Bull's conclusion was that I had probably received soft tissue damage, prevalent in whiplash accidents. Unfortunately, I had just gone through a long period of soft tissue healing and now I was back to square one.

When I first started in the life insurance business, an old-timer told me of a saying from the days of the Depression: "No man has the endurance of the man who sells life insurance." Over the years I often recalled that saying, and in my years in management I repeated it to many salespeople. Now I felt I was facing yet another endurance test and began to wonder if I had the strength to cope. It was like living in an eggshell or in a prison without bars. I was so fragile and had to be so careful with myself. There were so many restrictions and things I could not do or places I could not go. I was in dire straits, trying to manage and hold myself together while dealing with soft tissue damage, pinched nerve endings, and now a severe jolt to an area that had undergone a triple fusion. These were obvious areas of concern, but there was nothing anyone could do to help me. I just needed patience and time.

Before the accident in July 1991, we had planned to be in Hawaii for the month of October. Now it was September and we wondered if we should go ahead with our vacation. How could I go away on a holiday when I was so sick? I rationalized. "Yes, I am not well, but no, things will not be any different whether I am here or there. Yes, my wife deserves a much-needed break. Yes, my personal physician has given me his blessing as long as I am careful."

So I convinced myself and my wife that we should go, and go we did. The most difficult part of the trip was getting to and from the airports. The car's stopping and starting was nearly unbearable, but I had to endure it. We had a good vacation, if you could call it that, and after being away for a month I came home no different than when I left.

Because of this lack of progress, Dr. Bull felt maybe I should see Dr. May Ong, a specialist in pharmacology, to make sure we were not missing anything in my diagnosis or treatment. There was a six-month waiting period for appointments so I would not see this internist until early the next year.

In the meantime, I returned to the Thorson Rehabilitation Clinic not far from our old home in North Vancouver. Dr. Bull and I both hoped that one of the specialists at the clinic would be able to provide me with some relief from pain.

I had visited this clinic in 1989 for cortisone injections and biofeedback. Shortly after I started visiting the clinic again, Dr. Gordon Thorson, who was giving me cortisone injections in the neck area, suggested that I make an appointment with a specialist associated with the clinic who dealt with patients who had chronic pain problems.

I was impressed by this specialist as he questioned me at length on the nature of my problem, did an exhaustive medical examination, and made numerous measurements with a tape measure. He commented that I did not seem to have any identifiable neurological problems that might ultimately cause paralysis and added that my condition appeared to be benign, there was "no quick fix" for the problem, and it would require time to heal. Even then he could make no promises for a complete recovery. He prescribed a medication that I was on for a relatively short period of time. I later learned it was an anti-anxiety drug that could, in some cases, give relief from pain. In my case there was no change whatsoever, so the doctor discontinued it fairly soon. He recognized that my problem was not anxiety but pain, which I was dealing with as well as I could. He observed that I had learned to manage my problem well, but due to the recent setback I might need some additional help. Obviously I was not elated by his assessment as I was indeed looking for something much more concrete and a much quicker fix.

It wasn't till much later that I learned this "pain specialist" was a psychiatrist dealing in chronic pain rehabilitation. In an earlier chapter I mentioned that my personal physician thought the excruciating pain I was suffering could be "all in my head" and suggested I see a psychiatrist. I did not see one at that point, as the physical cause of my problem was discovered and I had my surgery. Now I had seen a psychiatrist and he concurred that my problem was not mental but physical pain.

This specialist recommended that I see a psychologist and that Sasha and I arrange to see a family counsellor at the clinic. He also said that I might benefit from some biofeedback sessions.

When Sasha and I met with the counsellor, I described how we coped individually and jointly with my ongoing problem. I reviewed how traumatic a setback the recent accident was for both of us in terms of my continued struggle with additional pain, the trauma I felt now when I was a driver or passenger in a vehicle, and my shyness and fear of the other driver. (I had not experienced this shyness after the original rear-ender, but the recent demolition derby left me with a lot of mistrust of other drivers.)

136

Sasha described how she had to adjust to a different lifestyle and outlined the amount of energy it had taken from her to care for me and my needs over a prolonged period of time. She explained how we had adjusted as much as possible to the circumstances, which we continued to cope with on a daily basis. She also talked about our move to the country and said it had been of benefit to her, allowing her to indulge her love of gardening and to enjoy the freedom and serenity we had in our new surroundings. She related how she watched me cope on a day-to-day basis as I tried to do tasks within my limitations, and she told how frightening it was to find me lying on the floor in various parts of the home. There were times when I would have to lie down where I was to get relief, even if I were outside. At other times I would lie down to watch an eagle soaring overhead as I could not bend my head backwards to look up without excruciating compounded pain.

I told the counsellor I would forfeit everything we had in return for my health status prior to the most recent accident. Then I reflected and amended that to say I would forfeit my half, leaving Sasha's to her, as I knew that I could get back to work. I had the capacity to rebuild whatever material possessions I had. But you cannot write a cheque in return for your health.

The counsellor was most impressed by the strength we had shown. In fact, she suggested I write a book on my experience. I told her that one of my goals was to write a book when I had recovered and I already had been keeping an extensive journal. She replied that based on what she had heard from both of us of our ability to gain enough strength and stamina from within, a written account could be of help to others.

In spite of her compassion, the counsellor openly admitted that she felt there was nothing she could do to help us. Her feeling was that we were handling the situation remarkably well. As the interview ended and we were leaving, she gave both Sasha and me a warm embrace and best wishes. I do not know if this was a typical ending to a session with this counsellor, but it was clear she had got caught up in the emotion of our situation and I give her points for her sincere concern and caring. This interview was a help in one sense, as it gave both Sasha and me an opportunity to express a lot of our feelings and dump our frustrations.

In early December I wrote in my diary, "I continue to be in much discomfort. Resting and meditating most of the day. As I look at the waterfall for a long period of time it has a mesmerizing, hypnotic effect. The shoulders, neck, skull continue to give me excruciating pain. My fingers are tingling in both hands, toes on right foot have needle-like feeling.

"Day to day continues to be an existence and I am in severe compounded pain. I continue to keep an open, positive mind, however, there are times when I begin to question the continuous positives I am feeding my mind, while seeing no progress healthwise. How can I keep telling myself I am getting better every day when it is not so? As strong as I am, I find it extremely difficult to live this type of prison-life lifestyle. I am damned if I partake in any type of activity and damned if I don't. Fragile as an eggshell and maybe even more so. The eggshell will crack and that's the end of it. My eggshell (head) continues to crack on a daily basis. It is a living hell."

It continued to be a difficult fight for my health. I told myself that prior to the second accident I had come a long way on the road to recovery. Now more than ever I must stick by my positive self-talk. If it had been a case of mind over matter, I would have had it beaten within days.

Because I had previously coped through very difficult times, I had developed a high tolerance for pain. A person who had never suffered pain as I had would have been seeing the doctor on a daily basis for relief, but doctors could not help besides prescribing medication. I would take the medication, though it did not seem to be making much difference. I rationalized that the pain would be much worse if I didn't take it. With rest and meditation I felt relief "beyond a tolerable level," but I was still in a lot of pain. I continued to have a positive attitude, but sometimes I wondered how much more of this my mind would accept.

These were difficult times for both Sasha and me, and it did not make things easier when she reminded me how difficult it was to live with a sick man. I knew she was right, but perhaps she did not know how difficult it was for me to live with myself and the condition I was in.

Early in January 1992 I had an appointment with the psychologist at the Thorson clinic. He recommended I attend a series of ten group sessions. At the same time I was in for each of these sessions, I would also be scheduled for biofeedback. He said he still had many pain-management techniques I had not tried and he hoped they would prove helpful, though he did stress that he had not yet reached the stage where he could have me walking over hot coals. He also recommended that I purchase from the clinic a book titled *The Chronic Pain Control Workbook*.

In spite of my adversity, living in the country was proving to be an enjoyable experience. On January 15, 1992, in our own yard, I picked a handful of pussy willows. No matter how sick you are, you can always receive great fulfillment from such an event. It is a kind of therapy. Perhaps the greatest satisfaction for me was to observe the smile on Sasha's face as she enjoyed seeing nature in bloom.

I started to read the *Chronic Pain Control Workbook* and picked out one interesting idea. It suggested that a person in pain could "put the pain on the shelf." I would try anything with imagery. What I did was put my pain in the medicine cabinet and close the door. Then I sealed the door with silicone and made sure there were no cracks. It was a great idea, but I found that when you are overwhelmed with pain it does not work. There was no way the silicone sealed the cracks.

Instead I waited for the biofeedback and group sessions to start on January 23, 1992.

Chapter 13

PAIN CLINIC

There are all kinds of management positions in almost every form of business. Then there is pain management, which is a twenty-four-hour-a-day vocation. In 1987, before my second surgery, my neurologist, Dr. Keyes, had encouraged me to attend sessions at a pain clinic. At that time I was in a great deal of pain, but it was also clearly recognized that my problem required surgery. In 1992 the only problem identified was that the July 1991 accident had been a serious setback. There was no indication that surgery was necessary. Instead, it was only a matter of time, waiting for the healing to take place if in fact it would.

The group sessions I was going to attend in 1992 were supposed to help identify areas of pain management I had not yet explored. I wasn't sure what these areas were as I had already been exposed to hypnosis, biofeedback, physiotherapy, the TENS machine, meditation, visualization, and other techniques. I decided to participate because I was desperate. All I had learned in pain management over the years was not working and neither was the medication. It was a major decision for me to attend these sessions, as it was an hour and a half drive to the clinic – and that was when road conditions were good – but I was not one to reject help. I told myself that I might well pick up some tips at these group sessions, something that would help me better manage my pain. As well, I had to take a positive attitude as I had in the past.

I arrived early for each group session so that I could fit in a biofeedback session with Lynda Thorson. This was not a new experience for me as I had previously attended a number of biofeedback sessions at the same clinic in 1989, after my second fusion surgery. The previous sessions put me in such a relaxed state that my eyelids would get heavy and I would fall asleep. This time, however, I met with no success. By the time I arrived at the clinic after the long drive I was in so much pain that this type of relaxation technique did nothing for me. The difference was that I had previously arrived at the clinic after a fifteen-minute walk that was relaxing rather than stressful.

I do believe that in the right set of circumstances, biofeedback can help restore the calm and serenity we all require and help the body in the healing process. It is an excellent relaxation technique. In fact, I acquired some tapes and videos of relaxing music, sounds, and images to play at home as a self-help. An added aspect of biofeedback sessions at the clinic was that as I listened to tapes or watched videotapes, I was wired up to a monitor that recorded such things as my pulse rate to track my response.

Feeling already drained from the drive, with no relief provided by biofeedback, I went on to group therapy. In the first session the psychologist gave an overview of the structure and purpose of the program. The group members introduced themselves and described their problems. I immediately wondered if I was in the right group, as many of the people didn't seem to be suffering from real physical pain but from problems of a different nature, many with some deep-rooted emotional causes. I decided that if the course continued this way it would, if nothing else, provide me with a study of humanity from a different perspective.

As the sessions progressed, various types of pain were covered: acute, chronic, organic, and physiological. The psychologist talked a lot about the stress-related causes of illness. He said that stress and anxiety supported pain and inhibited healing. I certainly could relate to part of this as I was under a lot of stress, but I could not understand how the stress would inhibit healing. For example, soft tissue damage takes a long time to heal whether you are under stress or not. I asked about this, but the psychologist would not answer questions of a medical nature.

He talked about how to interrupt the pain cycle and said that some type of sedative, such as an anti-depressant, could be prescribed for this. The psychologist also suggested breathing exercises, meditation, self-talk, positive thinking, visualization, self-hypnosis, and relaxation, but I was already practising all of these techniques. I was hungry for the unknown and the untried.

He spoke of anger and how it needed to be discharged. If anger was not discharged it would be bottled up and stored like poison.

Anger and depression were close cousins and both could hinder healing. This comment seemed appropriate, as I was finding that many of the participants felt a tremendous amount of anger, but in my opinion there was no one else in the group who was suffering from real pain as I was.

By real pain I mean pain that is emanating from a problem that requires attendance far beyond what medications can do. Medications may give some relief but they do not solve the problem.

I do not mean to say that the others in my group were not suffering from pain, as I believe pain can be described in much broader terms, including personal problems that have burdened the patient. What I found interesting was that such patients had lower levels of pain when they were on anti-depressants. It made me wonder if they were experiencing pain or if their problem was simply defined as such when in fact it was much more mind oriented. When I listened to the members of the group, I did not recognize the pain they were enduring.

I felt I was a mismatch in the group and to this day I wish it had not been so. I wish that I had been with a group of people who were suffering from the same kind of pain I was. With a sharing of ideas we could have helped each other – though this is not to say that individuals did not help others in the group I was in. I was still seeking that pain relief magic that I had not yet found. It could have come up at one of these sessions and I would always have wondered about that if I'd stopped attending.

This was both an enlightening and debilitating experience for me. Enlightening in that I was thrust into a group of people, not one of whom could relate to my problem. Moreover, because I decided to stay in the sessions I received a different perspective of life's difficulties and saw how other people are fighting for survival and looking for a healthy recovery.

The experience was debilitating because the three and a half hours of travel to and from the clinic would literally wipe me out. It would take me two or three days after a session to return to status quo. I would already be feeling compounded pain only twenty minutes after I'd left home on my way to the session. It was frightening, but I was glad I stayed with it. I had something to prove to myself. I had no regrets, but what a bear for punishment I was.

In retrospect, I found this an interesting sidetrack and an illumination of the medical search for answers. It was the psychiatrist who referred me to the psychologist after the prescription of anti-depressants made no difference to my condition. The psychologist, in turn, suggested I enroll in group therapy to learn how to better handle pain. The progression is interesting. If I had responded to anti-depressants, what direction would my treatment have taken? As well, I remember how my doctors had suggested before my second surgery that my pain was "all in my head." Had I seen a psychiatrist at that point, I likely would have ended up on anti-depressants even though my problem was physical pain, and surgery – and time – relieved it. I believe that there are doctors who do recognize real pain. I also believe that if I had not had a positive outlook on life, I could easily have fallen into the trap of treatment for multiple problems, one of which definitely would have been a serious case of depression.

Chapter 14

CONTINUING CHALLENGES

In late March 1992 I finally got in to see Dr. May Ong, the internist my personal physician suggested I see after the July 1991 accident. I'd had to wait six months for the appointment and in the meantime I'd gone through the pain clinic experience that left me no better off.

The doctor I saw now had a clinical degree in pharmacology, specializing in diagnosis and pain management. Dr. Bull felt I should see someone who focussed on pain management and who had some level of success in the field. Moreover, he was concerned that the accident might have caused some new problem that had not been recognized and for which I was not receiving treatment.

The words "pain management" were starting to sound like a worn-out record to me. With all I had been through and continued to go through, I felt I had earned a degree in pain management myself.

The internist discussed my medical history at length and did an examination. She noted I had damaged nerve roots, that the most recent accident was a serious setback, that there was a considerable amount of scar tissue from the surgery I had undergone, and that I did not appear to need further surgery.

We discussed medications and she suggested that an anti-seizure medication might be helpful for alleviating pain from the nerves that had been damaged. She commented that my personal physician already had me on medication from this family of drugs and complimented him for this.

She was most compassionate, recognizing the pain I was feeling and the fact that I had been forced to adjust to a new lifestyle, and she was pleased that I was attempting to lead as normal a life as possible, even though it was with a lot of difficulty and restrictions. She emphasized how important it was to be as mobile as possible under such duress and recognized I was doing everything possible in this area.

I described how I spent my days and how I had refrained from using the cervical collar, even though Dr. Bull suggested that I try wearing it while in a motor vehicle. I chose to endure the additional pain brought on by the stops and starts of driving, believing that the trade-off was a slow healing process as my neck muscles built up. She praised me for taking this attitude and agreed that wearing the collar would weaken my neck muscles as it had done in the past. She gave me a new prescription for anti-inflammatories that she felt might give me further relief. (Along with the change of medication, I now had to have periodic blood tests to make sure the drug was not harming vital organs – as if I were not already subjected to enough drugs and possible side effects.)

We discussed my recent attendance at the group therapy sessions and I told her they were of no help to me. She said that she also conducted such sessions and was associated with a pain clinic, but she recognized that further sessions of this type would be of no value to me. She scheduled a second appointment for me. Now that I was a patient, I was slotted for a six-week follow-up instead of the six-month wait I'd had before the initial appointment.

When I saw the internist again, we reviewed my progress and she increased the amount of medication I was taking and changed my sleeping-pill prescription. I had been on this pill for some time. One of its possible side effects was short-term memory loss and both my wife and I had noticed that I was having difficulty remembering certain things – nothing specific, but enough to be concerned.

I found the internist forthright and she didn't fudge when I asked her questions. The only answer that gave me some discouragement was her long-term prognosis. She said there was no quick fix and I might always have some residual problems. These would not keep me from leading a fairly normal life, but after all I'd been through it was hard to see such a long road still ahead.

Although I was doing everything within my power to restore my health, there was literally no progress. When you are suffering as I was and nothing is getting better, you cannot help but wonder whether there may be other aid that you have not yet sought. Specifically, I thought of the Mayo Clinic. Over the years I had often read of people who had gone to the Mayo Clinic for help. I actually knew a few personally. I thought of it as a last resort, and now it seemed to be time to make contact. I called the clinic's office in the U.S. to ask what procedure I must follow to set up an appointment. The person I spoke to said I would start by having a telephone interview with an evaluator who would take my health history. The clinic would look at this and decide what further action to take.

The person who did the phone interview took a detailed statement of my situation, cutting no corners, and told me that I would be contacted in a short while. Much to my surprise, I received a response promptly. It was not at all what I expected. I was told that after a careful review of the medical documentation, the doctors decided I was not a suitable candidate to seek help from the clinic. They felt there were highly skilled specialists in my geographical area who could treat my condition. I was disappointed, but I was also elated to have such a reinforcement that I was in good hands.

This is not to say I had questioned the medical help I was getting. There was no question I had faith in the practitioners looking after me, but I was getting restless and desperate, and when you see no positive change in your condition from month to month, it does become discouraging.

After such a prolonged period of disability I had learned many techniques for gaining some relief from pain. I would sit upright in a high-back chair with a small, soft pillow at the back of my neck, staying in this position for hours on end and trying to move my head as little as possible. With every movement of my head, whether it was up and down or sideways, I had extreme compounded pain radiating to the skull.

I would meditate in this position, do self-hypnosis, rest, or watch the cascading waterfall until it mesmerized me. Occasionally I saw a moving shadow across the treetops and then I would go out to the patio to watch the eagle soar. It is incredible how much you will see pass by when you are sitting still.

Our home was on a migration route for hummingbirds. We kept three feeders stocked for these birds at all times, and from my high-back chair I could watch them for hours. They are marvels of nature and their speed and ability to maneuver make them a sight to behold. Their colouring is forever changing in the sunlight and shadows.

It was important to learn to live with a painful, crippling disability, but it was even more important not to allow the disability to destroy me or to prevent my maintaining interests and activities within my capabilities. I refused to become bedridden or feel sorry for myself. I did, however, with much resistance, accept the fact that I needed a medicine bottle and a lot of bed rest to help me keep going. I would have done anything for a day of good health.

In spite of living in what I called paradise, my days were filled with pain. It was difficult. I was an adult and yet I had trouble bending over to tie my shoes. If I had the strength to make myself breakfast, I'd be in compounded pain simply from mixing a bowl of porridge. I'd bend over to fill the gas tank on the lawn mower and the result would be severe compounded pain radiating to the skull. Many times I wondered if this was the same old problem or if it was something new. If it were new, maybe I needed immediate medical attention. I would always resort to more rest and relaxation (as if I had not had enough of it), things would settle down, and I knew that had I gone to the doctor, there would have been nothing he could do. I always hoped and prayed that I would not make the wrong judgment call when I should have sought medical attention, but I had learned the symptoms of my condition well and the best way to handle them.

Anyone who is confronted with a problem that requires time and a great deal of patience can adapt, but it takes a strong will and the power of mind over matter to hold yourself together and make the best of a given situation. It takes willpower and lots of it, hourly, daily, weekly, monthly...sometimes for years as it was in my case. Although it would have been easy, I would not crawl into a corner and feel sorry for myself. I was in a "Damned if you do and damned if you don't" situation. I had to learn to do what I could without hurting myself further, be satisfied with that, and forget about the rest.

I think we take good health for granted. We have trouble believing - or don't want to admit – there are forces that can overpower us and leave us helpless. I know that when I was stricken, I still couldn't understand how the pain had so much power over me. All I could do was try to manage the pain on a day-to-day basis. Such pain causes a total redirection of your life into uncharted waters. There is no such thing as prior planning for this kind of event. It is frightening and it is stressful. However, if you use all of your God-given resources to the fullest, you will survive the change.

I found the saying "If it is going to be, it is up to me" gave me strength, though it is important to be able to recognize what is up to you and what is up to the medical professionals helping you if you are dealing with a medical problem. Repeating this phrase helped me rise to many occasions, even ones that may have been strenuous for a healthy individual. For example, in late May 1992 I was asked to be master of ceremonies for the wedding of one of my nieces. I had the privilege of being MC at previous weddings, but these were occasions when I was healthy, not in a state where I couldn't know what my health might be on the day of the wedding. Nevertheless, I consented.

When the wedding day came, as with most of my days, I was not feeling too well. When I bent my neck to look down I had compounded pain in my skull, and I wondered how I would manage at the podium. When I arrived at the hall, the first thing I did was seek out the manager and ask him to show me the podium. With some quick improvising he was able to raise its height so that I did not have to bend my head as much. The time came for the ceremonies and I was well prepared, surprisingly calm, and everything went off without a hitch. At the end of the day I was wiped out, but only my wife and I knew it and I had a great feeling of satisfaction. I had proved to myself that I could still stand a challenge. The big gamble was that I did not know in advance whether it was within my limitations. But then, isn't life about facing up to the challenges of the day and making the most of them?

I had learned many ways to manage with my problem. If I wanted to see something off to the side, rather than turning my head I would turn my whole body. To tie my shoes I would lift my foot to a chair. When I made porridge for breakfast I would not bend my head downward to watch. I would use a face cloth to wash my face after shaving rather than bending over to wash. If I had to pick something up I would crouch rather than bend over. I learned to be protective and guard myself where I could to avoid added pain. No one ever asked me why I was squatting when I was filling the gas tank on the car, though I can recall some strange looks coming my way. It was not easy to become alert to potential stresses and adjust to them, as I had never had to do this before.

When my new drivers licence arrived in the mail, Sasha took one look at the photo and stated, "In the last year you have aged ten years. You look like a man of seventy." The comment was not solicited, but I was glad she expressed how she saw me. Obviously the trauma of the past year had taken its toll. My only hope was that I still had the years of a sixty-one-year-old left in me.

Towards the end of June I saw the internist again. We reviewed my ongoing problems, the medications I was taking, and the difficulty I had getting rest at night. She was most understanding and assured me that things would settle down with time. She also said that at this stage she felt it important that I start an exercise program. I would start with two exercises. In one I would sit in a high-back armchair with a pillow behind my head and push my head backwards into the pillow (head retraction). In the second I would lie on my back on the floor with arms outstretched at my sides, then swing both arms up beside my head.

I reminded her that any type of physio I'd done in the past had always ended up being regressive, and I could not help recalling the comment of Dr. B when, exasperated by the deterioration in my condition after physiotherapy and exercises, he said, "Why don't they just leave you alone to heal?" I did not mention this to Dr. Ong.

She in turn asked me if I was maybe being "gun shy." I assured her I was not and said she would have my utmost cooperation, as I would do anything to get better. I also pointed out that the fact I refused to use the cervical collar for certain activities since the July 1991 accident showed I was not "gun shy." I was, on a daily basis, carrying my head on my own and rotating it as much as possible. I was always a believer in "No pain, no gain" and was testing myself constantly.

The exercises she was prescribing were new. I had not done any like them in the past, so I thought maybe they'd be beneficial. I immediately started the prescribed program. By the end of the first day I was feeling additional compounded pain. I thought it could be the result of the previous day's travel, as this was a common experience. Two days later, however, I was in such extreme pain that I went to see Dr. Bull. I told him there were no changes in what I was doing except for the introduction of the exercise program. He suggested I discontinue it immediately and get in touch with the internist.

Unfortunately it was the beginning of a weekend, so I had to wait it out before I could talk to Dr. Ong.

It was a hard situation for me. I was in worse pain than I had been a few days earlier and the regression was self-inflicted. Though I had discontinued the exercises, the pain was getting progressively worse. It was obvious I was not ready for an exercise program to strengthen my muscles. Even an activity as simple as shaking the hummingbirds' sugar and water solution in a container left me in unbearable pain from the neck radiating to the skull, arms, and shoulder.

As I thought about how things had changed so quickly from bad to worse, I knew I had not been "gun shy," but I was paying the price of being caught in a "Damned if you do and damned if you don't" situation. I was suffering the consequences of "doing," but if I hadn't done the exercises I would have wondered if they might have helped me. As well, the setback would let the internist know where I was at.

To do or not to do

When we are not well we have more time on our hands than we would ever have thought possible. Unfortunately, this type of time can drag on and on and on. We need this time, lots of it, in order for our body to heal. However, if we can provide some balance of activity and rest to help fill in that time, we will enjoy a better lifestyle, even though we are overwhelmed with trauma. Doing something may take away some of this burden of pain and trauma we are living – or existing – with.

Before we moved to the country I created a list of things I wanted to do on the new property. I was excited by the possible rehabilitation activities it offered. I had used project lists while in business and found I could not work without them. Moreover, once I had put something in writing I did not have to keep it in my memory bank. And because ideas are fleeting, I often found that I would forget an excellent idea if I didn't write it down because it would be pushed out of my mind by all the other thoughts and ideas I had to keep track of.

During my illness, this "I can/I want to do" list helped me keep going. Instead of having to think of something to do, I could pick a project at any time. I found there was a right time and a wrong time for certain projects. Some of them were beyond my physical capability at one moment, but well within my limits later. I kept adding to the list and now it is so long that I know I could not accomplish everything on it in my lifetime. All of the activities listed are of interest to me. All are things I would like to try someday.

So long as activities were within my capabilities and did not cause undue pain or regression, everything I did helped to maintain my interest in life and often heightened my desire to get better. My activities had a calming effect and diverted my mind from the pain (mind over matter). At times I would ask myself if I were causing more pain, but I would usually have a good sense of my limitations and not push beyond them. And the resulting feeling of accomplishment gave me great satisfaction.

The various forms of activity I used were not pain-relieving techniques, they were not the answer to my problems. Rather, they proved to be a form of escape that allowed me to carry on, continuing to suffer from excruciating pain but under a different set of circumstances. In a situation like mine, a person needs diversion from the real problem. Although I will be the first to admit it is difficult and requires a high degree of discipline, it is also doable. It may be that you are unable to do too much, but remember the old saying, "By the inch, it's a cinch." It will give you the spirit and momentum to carry on.

I do not know how I managed except for the fact that I would not give up. It takes a lot of tenacity to keep going, especially when you have so little encouragement from the medical profession on whom you are totally reliant. I am sure that I would not have survived if it were not for my activities and hobbies. I also did many things during the ten-year period that I would not likely have done under normal circumstances.

During my darkest days, when I was unable to start any projects, I was still able to remain active in a restricted manner. I made up my mind that the last thing I would carve out of my life was my Commitment to Health walking program. In the course of a day I would rest and walk, rest and walk too many times to mention. However, what a sense of achievement it was! I hoped it would be a means of escape from pain. That was not to be, but it did give me a break from being a total prisoner in my own home, and it gave me the opportunity to meet and exchange pleasantries with many fine people in our neighbourhoods. Again, I strongly suggest that anyone with a problem or a multitude of problems should start the walking activity as a priority activity if they are able to do so. Start slowly, without covering too great a distance at first, increasing your distance progressively, always remembering that you do have time on your hands.

When you are faced with a prolonged disability, even though you are living with the outside world you are effectively living in a world of your own. This world you must rethink, reshape, remold to fit your environment and your capabilities. You must rethink your values, the importance of family, friends, work, and other ways of being an asset to society. It is imperative that you not think any less of yourself as a human being. You must allow yourself time to refocus some of your priorities, as presently you are no doubt majoring on the biggest concern in your life – your health. (In other cases the concern could be a relationship, your business, or your work.) I am not saying that you should not focus on what is causing your problem, but you must accept that beyond certain boundaries there is nothing more you can do, and past that point you must work to get on with life as best you can and create other interests. This is not an easy task, but when you look at the alternatives it is a choice of regression or progression. I have made it crystal clear which path I chose to follow. Not everyone can do it on their own, but I believe we have enough qualified care to help people who choose progression.

I was fortunate to have the ability to rationalize, think things through, put them in perspective, and set up a game plan. It did not happen overnight, but it did happen, under the most difficult conditions. The secret was to have an open, inquiring mind and do all I could within my limited range of ability.

If you have not been involved in any type of hobby or activity, it is important first to identify the degree of your mobility and your capabilities. Having done that, start a list of things you would like to do. It is critical that as soon as an idea comes to mind you write it down. As I said above, once you have written down an idea it is out of your mind in a sense and leaves you wide open for the exploration of yet other new ideas.

You can only do one thing at a time and it is important to remain goal-oriented in this regard. Focus on the project at hand. It is easy to find that where you had nothing to do, you are now overwhelmed with projects, so much so that you could feel they are not worthwhile. When you have been down and out and you allow your creative mind to start charting your future, you may feel you cannot handle the load. Start with the simplest of projects, a day at a time, and then allow others into your daytime activity as both time and ability permit. It takes a lot of courage to get started and also to carry on.

As time goes on you may find you quickly adapt and bring things to completion, depending on the size of the project. At other times you may find you will skip a day or two, or work on multiple projects, which may help avoid boredom. Boredom is a sickness we must avoid. Boredom can only help you regress. We have to take the letters d-o-m out of the word and BORE on with positive, health-building activities. If I could do it, so can you, but in order to do it you must make a start, if necessary a bit at a time. It matters not how small the daily bits are at the initial stages. What matters is the bit.

It took me a tremendous amount of patience to do something over a long time, particularly when my negative self-talk reminded me how quickly I would have finished the activity had I been healthy. However, what at one time would have been very important became secondary in importance, and as time went on I became both pleased and amazed at how much I could accomplish doing a little every day, no matter how little, over long periods of time. Through self-talk of "Rome was not built in a day," I was able to tone down the negatives and have a great sense of accomplishment with every completed project.

If you are faced with a disability of some kind, get that pencil and paper right now, stop reading this book, and jot down those hot ideas of things to do. If you are in any type of situation where you can see this type of planning could be helpful to you, take the time to create a To Do list. It could change your direction in life. It did mine.

Perhaps even more importantly, if you know of someone who you think could benefit from my pencil and paper philosophy, share it with them now. Stop reading, pick up the phone, and call them, NOW. Both you and they will be glad you did. It is hard to believe what a sense of direction a pen and a piece of paper will give. It may change your life for the better.

My comments in this chapter apply to everyone, in all walks of life, bar none. I am coming at this from the perspective of someone who has experienced ten years of unbelievable pain and disability, but the needs of disabled people are, for the most part, the same as those of society in general. The difference is that the lives of people with disabilities have been disrupted to such an extent that they may require a lot of care (and no matter what the extent and nature of the disability, they must not give up). But anyone can have problems, anyone can need activities to distract them from the day-to-day burdens of life. This often becomes an issue in retirement, for example. All too often when people reach the point of retirement they regress because they do not know what to do with themselves. They have too much time on their hands and no interests to keep them busy. If you are reading this book and are near – or even years from – retirement, start your list of "Things To Do In Retirement."

Now I have an endless list of things I want to do, and the list keeps growing. Many are things I did not do earlier because they were beyond my capability as far as my health was concerned. Although on one hand I find it strange that I have such a desire to plan things to do in the future, on the other hand I feel as if I am compensating for ten lost years. I do not see myself ever being in a position where I will not be doing something or will not have something planned to do within my capabilities.

Chapter 15

FACET JOINTS

I spent the weekend sitting totally still, with no head movement for hours on end. At this stage my biggest hope was that I would be able to return to my condition of only a few days before. When I finally reached the internist by telephone and told her what had happened in the short time since I saw her, the response was instant. She said I did not have a muscle problem as that would not have produced such quick regression. She stated it was a facet joint and ligament problem.

This new diagnosis hit me like a ton of bricks. After all the problems I had gone through, I was now confronted with some new and totally foreign medical terminology. Dr. Ong said I should have a facet block, a procedure she described as an injection into the facet joint under X-ray. It would be done by a specialist in a hospital on an outpatient basis. The internist said she would arrange for me to have this procedure done.

I was caught by surprise and I immediately questioned the advisability of my seeing yet another specialist, especially since, as I understood it, the procedure she was advising me to have was an invasive one. The internist understood my apprehension and said she would see me first and explain my new problem and its treatment in detail; then we could arrange to have the facet block performed.

This was not a happy day. Here I was in much worse shape than I had been just days ago, and now I was dealing with a new problem. I didn't even know what a facet joint was.

On the other hand, I could not help but think of my philosophy of "If it's broken, fix it." After a few months of non-manipulative treatment, the internist, with an attempt at an exercise program, had identified the root of my problem. I remembered that my personal physician had sent me to this internist to make sure he had not missed another problem. Dr. Bull had made the right call.

Dr. Ong changed my anti-inflammatory medication in hopes that a different prescription would lessen the facet joint pain. This did give me a little relief - and when you are suffering severe pain, a little relief is a lot. I also found that the sleeping pills were helping. I was sleeping well. The night is short when you are sleeping well, but when you are not sleeping well, when you are tossing and turning, the night goes on forever, painful and disturbing. And when you are not sleeping, the body is not getting as much time for healing.

Every day I made notes in my diary of my activities and health. I felt a great sense of relief when I put what I was feeling to paper. On occasion Sasha would read my notes for the day and her tears would flow as she read. Around this time I asked Sasha how much of a burden I was to her. She replied that she worried a lot when she saw the state I was in and that she felt helpless and wished she could do more for me. She also said that she was doing her best not to intrude on me, to protect me yet not treat me as if I were disabled.

When someone is close to you and caring for you, he or she can unknowingly start caring for you as if you are an invalid when in fact you are not. This is not to say I did not need a lot of help and support, but it was important that I was self-sufficient. I did not wish to be treated as someone who needs help with every move. All I wanted was to manage myself as best I could under the circumstances and to lead as normal a life as possible. It was a difficult period for both of us and I often thought about how the vows of marriage led to a lot of unknowns.

At the end of July 1992 I wrote in my notes that because I had received such severe setbacks from simple head movement, I would never again submit to any type of exercise involving head movement. If asked to do so, I would resist. I had suffered enough. Having put this in writing, it was a commitment etched in stone. I decided that if I was to heal, I would do so under the guidance of nature. I would continue to do everything within my power and capabilities to help the healing process, but I also began to ask myself if I had maybe plateaued and if this was where I would be for the rest of my life.

I had come a long way in learning how to manage and not self-destruct. However there were certain activities that I considered to be within my capabilities that did set me back. Driving or being a passenger in a vehicle was always a setback, but I rationalized that unless I made a start in building my muscles up, they would never recover. This was a dramatic illustration of a "Damned if you do and damned if you don't" predicament.

In mid-August I saw the internist and we reviewed my progress and the medications I was taking. She showed me a booklet that illustrated the spinal column and the location of the facet joints (see "A brief introduction to the spine" in Chapter 1). No one I talked to outside the medical profession had ever heard of a facet joint. Now I learned that each facet joint links two vertebrae together. They are small joints made up of cartilage surrounded by tough fibres and are located at the back of the vertebra. These joints are movable, like the knee, and allow the spine to flex. In a facet block, cortisone is injected into the joint. If this relieved the symptom of pain, it was an indication that the problem was indeed caused by the facet joint.

I learned that because my spine was fused at three levels, all the stress of whiplash from the most recent accident had been placed on the areas above and below the area that was fused. The problem was to determine where most of the damage was and this was where the facet block procedure would help. Because the pain had increased when I attempted exercises and because the anti-inflammatory medication was helping somewhat, the internist came to the conclusion that the problem was at the cervical 2/3 level, but she emphasized that she could not be sure and the problem might be at other levels.

The facet blocks would be performed at various levels, starting at the 2/3 level, to pinpoint the problem area. I would undergo a series of blocks at two-week intervals. Dr. Ong told me that the cortisone injection was not harmful as long as I was not given too much cortisone. She also said that I should have immediate relief after the procedure, though there could be a little discomfort for a few days.

At this time I questioned whether, seeing as how the anti-inflammatory medication was helping a little, we should give it more time to work. The internist agreed and we decided that if there was no further progress after twelve weeks on medication, facet blocks would be done.

The prolonged, severe pain was difficult to control, and my blood pressure had gone up again due to the extreme stress. I continued to do everything I could to control the pain, but it was a force unto itself. Suffering with pain for such a long time gives you cause to question:

Will I ever heal? Will I ever get back to work? Will I have to have someone care for me forever? Will I always be living within certain limitations? Why are we so advanced that we can send a man to the moon and yet not have the answers for many medical concerns? Why, why, why?

Anyone plagued with problems of any type will ask such questions, especially when the problems are medical. We spend such large sums of money on research in virtually every field of medicine, yet there are many unanswered questions and missing solutions. Much of our knowledge only arises in response to problems. For example, I believe that we might not have learned all we have about the skeleton if it had not been for our two- and four-wheeled vehicles. It was the accidents on the highways and byways that caused so many crippling situations and encouraged us to find out how all the muscles, nerves, and the spine are connected. In a split second human beings may find themselves confined to a wheelchair for the rest of their lives. Cartilage and ligaments, once damaged, are slow to recover if they ever do, and here I was with nerve root, facet joint, cartilage, ligament, and muscle damage, bone spurs, scar tissue, and stress beyond compare.

How do you deal with such a host of problems and make the best of each and every day? It takes guts, the will to live, faith in self and others, a lot of fight, and the endurance to keep pushing forward when the walls seem to be caving in all around you. To keep climbing that mountain, reaching for that peak while continually slipping backwards, takes a great deal of inner strength. One foot forward and two feet backwards makes for a long climb.

I received accolades from many people for my ability to cope. While they had admiration for my ability to manage, I was burning with envy, wishing I was out there pursuing my career as they were.

Learning to live with severe pain on a day-to-day basis was most debilitating. It would have been so easy to feel sorry for myself and give up. It may have been the easy way to go, but I was determined to do something every day, no matter how insignificant it may have been at the time. And the ability to say I did something in my restricted way of life meant a lot to me. I was constantly reaching out and testing my abilities only to learn that nothing was changing. More than ever I recognized that if I was going to heal, it would take time.

I saw Dr. Bull every month and on numerous occasions I tried to put myself in his shoes and wondered how difficult it must be for him to be so limited in what he could do for me. I admired the tenacity with which he continued to cope with me. One area that I found difficult to understand was the medical profession's inability to give me a definitive answer on when I might get back to work. Originally I was to be off for a few months after surgery. Months turned into years, then there was another major setback, and now here I was yearning to get back to what I left behind.

In late September I had an appointment with the internist. She reviewed the medications I was taking and was pleased when I told her that the severity of pain in the morning had eased up a little (by evening it was status quo). This was apparently a good sign, though it was hard for me to appreciate the improvement when I remained in constant pain.

We discussed how little progress there had been in the six weeks since my previous appointment and I told her that in retrospect I realized I should have consented to having the facet blocks done then rather than waiting to see what results the medication would have. Her surprising and interesting response was that she does not push her patients. I wondered whether I should have been more aggressive. Usually my attitude is that when a problem is identified and needs to be fixed, it should be fixed immediately. Before my fusion surgeries I had to wait many months to see specialists for their expert opinions, even though I believed surgery was my only solution. Though I respect an expert opinion, the wait at that time had caused me to deteriorate considerably before I finally had the surgery, which should have occurred immediately. At that time I had been a zombie, totally reliant on the medical profession. This time I was the one who suggested we take a wait-and-see approach and give time and medication a chance to help. There is, however, a big difference between six weeks and years of waiting.

The internist gave me the name of the neuroradiologist who would do the facet blocks and told me the procedure would take place at St. Paul's Hospital in Vancouver. Someone at the hospital would call and tell me the time and date when I should come in.

In early October 1992 I made the following entry in my diary: "What is not comforting is the level of pain I have in the neck area, just from writing these notes. This is where I am at, it matters not what I do, something or nothing. I still have to hold my head up."

And that was the difficulty – holding my head up. One of the things I became conscious of was how much we move our heads and flex our necks. When I was talking to someone, I would observe that person's head movements. It is incredible how many times in a short period of time, a sentence or two, people will nod their heads. We take it for granted, yet here I was in compounded pain with every movement of my head. I was so aware of how easily I could hurt myself that it became second nature to turn my whole body when necessary and avoid any head nodding. I suppose this was a part of pain management and by now I was skilled at avoiding pain if I could help it. The "No pain, no gain" philosophy certainly did not apply here. I learned how important it was to have a healthy neck. It must carry the weight of the head - approximately fourteen pounds.

I was in a catch twenty-two situation. No matter what I did or did not do, I was subjected to neck pain radiating to the skull. I was damned if I did – even subdued, restricted, controlled, guarded activity caused some pain – and damned if I did not – inactivity would leave my muscles weak. For example, you might think attending a three-hour live theatre performance would be good for me and no strain on my neck. Such events were indeed great outings, but the deep vise-grip of pain in my neck radiating to my skull as I held my head upright would distract me so much that all I could do was squirm in my seat in a vain attempt to find a more comfortable position. Only people who have experienced or are presently experiencing such pain could understand what I am relating. Others may wonder why I would put myself in these situations if it hurt so much, but had I not partaken in activities within my limitations I was "Damned if you don't," as I would never have restored the neck muscles.

There were other advantages to these outings. Social activity helped me keep my mental faculties working and it was therapeutic to hear Sasha laughing at a humorous play. There were times when laughter was a precious commodity. Whenever possible I would try to turn a stressful situation to laughter. It can be done and it must be done if both the caregiver and the recipient are to maintain a healthy mental balance.

"If it is going to be, it is up to me." How many times have I shared these words with others and on a daily basis with myself? The problem now was that I was limited in helping myself. All I could do was manage the pain and hold myself together. During this traumatic period I could not get inside and fix the problem. I was also beyond the reach of further medical help, except for the medication that offered some measure of relief. (Of course I always wondered what effect this medication was going to have on me in the long term.)

I continued to be in a "fight or flight" predicament and I was determined to keep fighting. At least the medication kept me at a plateau. I was having days I would refer to as "better" and "fair," though always I would be back to the familiar compounded pain by the end of the day. I continued to test myself. If my test proved to be too much activity I would end up for a week at home, practising my pain-management techniques, while the settling process returned me from severe pain to the status quo.

By late October, a month after telling the internist I would go ahead with the facet blocks, I had still not been called for the procedure. I called the office of the internist and explained to the receptionist that I had no response from the hospital and I was wondering what the time frame might be before I would be called.

The receptionist said she would check into the matter and get back to me. Within the hour she phoned back and said the hospital had done a thorough check and had lost the first requisition. She assured me that another requisition had already been completed and said that had I not called, I might have ended up waiting a long time.

Within days I had a call confirming that my first facet block was scheduled for November 3, 1992. How time flies when you are not well. Eight months after seeing the internist, and after much suffering, I was scheduled for yet another invasive procedure.

Keeping up with living

Had my life been taken up 100 percent with my problem, day in and day out without any other interests, I have no doubt that it would have finished me off. There is no question that I was overwhelmed

163

with pain so strong that I would have run away and hid if I could. However, I knew this was not something I could run away from. I had to deal with it head on and this is what I did to the best of my capabilities.

I had never had so much free time, but I had also never been so restricted in what I could or could not do. These limitations were not imposed by the medical profession; they were imposed by my body. I discovered there is not a stronger force around. When my body said jump, I did not say how high; I immediately lay down. Pain did not want an hour or two of my time daily; it wanted me twenty-four hours a day, but I vowed to have some of that time to myself. I learned how best to react, how to respond, and how to manage when I had overdone it, which was all too easy to do. And I continued to maintain my hobbies and activities between visits with the medical profession and the time-outs my body called for me every day.

From the day I was rear-ended in November 1984, my life started to change. It was slow, subtle, and painful and I soon found that in addition to my deteriorating health condition, my way of life was deteriorating as I was not able to participate in some of the activities that had become a part of my life.

Swimming was out. Tennis – forget it. Bowling was a disaster. Cycling was now a dream. And cross-country skiing was no longer for me. Dining and dancing had become dining with no dancing. The real world had disappeared and the world of function-if-you-can was setting in.

I was a person of great determination. Faced with something new in my life, I just wanted to get to the root of my problem, resolve it, and get on with life. This philosophy was sound and simple in the business world, but not so simple in the world of health and recovery. There were suddenly many obstacles in my way and many questions - will I recover, will I be crippled, how long will it take to recover, will I ever again have some level of good health? The good old days were well in the past.

The adjustment from an active life, getting up every morning and going to work, to a life of coping with a debilitating health condition was a tough one. I had a new full-time job – fighting for survival – for which I had no training. Apprenticing in this new field was not only difficult but also distasteful. I had not applied for this job, did not want it, yet I was locked into it for an unspecified time frame.

I was aware that it was important for Sasha and me to get away from it all – including the pain – periodically, even if only for a few hours. In everyday life going to a movie, a concert, or a live play is taken for granted, just another outing dependent on one's tastes. In my situation, all these activities, which had been a way of life for Sasha and me prior to my injury, took on a totally different and special meaning. Initially they were rare and painful – so painful that I often questioned why I went. When I did go, it was out of a sense of duty to Sasha. This may seem puzzling as she was the one arranging for the tickets, doing the driving, persevering with me. It might seem that all the duty was hers. But I was able to see the enjoyment and fulfillment the performance gave her and realized it was worth her arranging and my pain. Even though we were both totally engrossed in my health problem, we were only two of many in the audience and our problems were no more or less important than anyone else's. I must say, I came to have a much deeper appreciation for those who were in wheelchairs at such events.

During the summers, Sasha and I would get away for a day to the city or the ocean. Once we took a three-day trip to the Gulf Islands. Each and every activity brought me great stress, but I vowed to do them and carry on as best I could. It was important to get out for a few hours, a day if possible, or even a few days. When you are confined close to home, it is hard to believe how much it means to get away for even a few hours. This was especially necessary for Sasha. I could not allow her to be totally swallowed up in my problems. There were times when I was at my worst and Sasha was overwhelmed. Somehow we were always able to recognize these situations and not only discussed them but agreed that Sasha should take a break for a day or a few days. Unfortunately, there were no breaks for me.

One activity that had become a part of my life prior to the accident was my Commitment to Health aerobic walking program. As I've said before, this discipline of walking was an important part of my daily routine and in spite of the skull pain that increased with every step, I carried on with it. In fact, with my days stretching empty before me, the walking became a high priority for filling that time and I found it nourished my body, mind, and soul.

We had friends over, spreading out these visits so I didn't get worn out, and although I may not have been the best of hosts, I did my best to participate in each visit. All too often I would spend the better part of the visit sitting in a high-back chair with pillow support, but it was better to be visiting than drowning in my sorrows. You do not need guests every day, but a variety of people to talk to keeps your mind active and entertained.

Rest and relaxation had taken on a new meaning as well, though I was not trained to do them on a full-time basis. I found that I had a lot of time for reading, but it's hard to fill each and every day with rest, walking, relaxation, reading, and visitors. I started to think about how I could fill in some of the spare hours.

During my adult life I did not have a hobby as such, as raising two daughters and four sons took all my non-working time. As a family we were never short of activities, and I could easily say that my family was my hobby. I always intended to develop other interests when I had the time, but I hadn't expected that time to come so soon.

I have already mentioned some of the activities I pursued, especially after we moved to the country – rebuilding the log cabin on our property, gardening, and overseeing the restoration of antique vehicles. There are so many things one can start doing to help make a brighter day. I also became interested in native artwork after one of our sons told me of a friend who was a painter. I met this man, Wilfred Baker from the Capilano Indian reserve, and he offered to bring some of his work for me to see. I was so impressed by his traditional native images that I found myself commissioning him to do a painting of an eagle for me. It was completed, delivered to our home, and a new collection was started. Wilfred introduced me to Stewart Jacob, an artist who worked in pottery. I admired his beautiful clay bowls with engraved and painted masks, eagle heads, sea serpents, fish, and whales and I have acquired a varied collection of handcarved works over many years.

To watch a skilled artist craft a piece from a block of wood is an inspiring sight. The carving is not done from a detailed set of blueprints. Instead, it arises from the imprint on the mind of the carver.

Although the purchase of a new piece is a fleeting experience, the work itself is a lovely and living memento each and every day thereafter. There is a spiritual element as well. Touching one of these objects on a given day can send shivers down my spine and inspires me.

Another therapeutic activity is creating objects for yourself. It is often not too expensive to buy the raw materials and then you have the fulfillment of crafting an item and enjoying it. In my case, I have been an amateur photographer for many years. I have yet to upgrade my skills with classroom instruction, but I have taught myself enough to produce some nice photographs. Whether they are spring, summer, fall, or winter scenes, storm clouds or the sun setting, each and every one tells a story. I end up with many of the same settings but never the same picture. A memory may fade or be forgotten, but capturing a scene on a photograph provides a life-long living memory. I can take many memories on one roll of film and it is not an expensive hobby. As well, this activity takes me on an adventure hunt as I look for that interesting snapshot.

Our children visited during all the holidays seasons, and every time we saw the grandchildren they had grown some more. We made family outings to nearby lakes, golf driving ranges, or other recreational centres. When the grandchildren visited, I spent as much time with them as I could, taking them out for sledding, skiing, ice skating, road hockey, bowling, swimming, hiking in the woods, a game of hide and seek with the dog, go-carts, water slides, tennis, movies, a hockey game, a drive in an old vehicle, a ride on the tractor, a visit with great-grandmother, a game of cards, checkers, or pool, or an expedition into the woods the old-fashioned way to bring out a Christmas tree. After taking the grandchildren for an outing there was always a pit stop for hamburgers, pizza, ice cream, or some other treat. I liked to get away with them for a few hours so I could get to know them. Because I was unable to travel to their homes, I wanted to share time and activities with them that they could remember.

One year we spent a day at the Pacific National Exhibition, Vancouver's agricultural fair, where the Ukrainian community was celebrating its 100th anniversary in Canada. The exhibits, and the chance to speak to the exhibitors and volunteers in our mother tongue, were heartwarming. The displays showing what the pioneers of the community went through when they settled in Canada reminded me of stories my aunt used to tell me of her arrival in Canada in the early 1900s. Her first home was a dugout in the ground. She had a woodstove for cooking and heating. Her son was a milkman who would take me out on his rounds delivering milk with a horse and buggy. In the cold of winter, milk delivery was tricky. As the milk froze and expanded, a milk and cream icicle erupted from the bottle, raising the cap from the rim of the bottle mouth. My cousin left the bottles on the doorstep with the cap sitting precariously on top of this icicle. In turn, this reminded me of how I would play hockey in the thirties. Even though times were tough, all the boys seemed to have ice skates and hockey sticks. We would make homemade pucks. How do you make a hockey puck? We would follow the horses as they made their way through the streets in the cold of winter. When the horse had to defecate we would make a dash for the spoils. We took the horse dung, shaped it into a hockey puck, and in no time at all it was frozen and ready for use. The pucks would break up if we hit them too hard, but there were always more where they came from.

Memories are what life is made of and anyone who is bothered by bad memories should do some soul clearing. Bad memories alone may put you in a state of ill health. Let the good memories overrule the bad. A positive side-effect of many of my projects and activities was the creation of new, good memories.

Positives that help you use time are priceless. Granted, anything we do today seems to require money. But if you are not well, it also takes money to keep you in medication. The difference is that the money you spend on medication may only help you to better manage on a day-to-day basis. The money you spend on a project within your means will give you something you can look at, touch, and feel good about forever. This sense of gratification, of accomplishment, adds to your self-worth. No one can do what you can do but you. We could feel sorry for ourselves and spend nothing other than for the necessities of life. Conversely, we can start on small projects within our means and capabilities and probably not have too serious an impact on our financial resources. And such activities are probably the cheapest medication money will buy. The secret is to do it.

I learned how important it is to maintain or develop interests and hobbies, even though I was suffering from a prolonged health problem. They were a diversion, something to keep my mind stirred up. It is vital to keep an active mind. My orthopaedic surgeon would always say "use it or lose it" in reference to my neck problem. I firmly believe that this is also the case with the brain. If you are constantly using it, you stay razor sharp. It is amazing how the more information you feed it, the more it will take. It is also amazing that if you do not use that information, it will be put aside for future recall. My brain power helped me through difficult periods, and maintaining mental activity was beneficial.

I will readily admit that had I been well, I may never have done some of the things I ended up doing during my rehabilitation process. There were things I wanted to do eventually, after I retired, but I never thought I'd get to some of them, as well as new interests, during a period of disability.

Anyone can develop their own activities and hobbies. There is an endless supply of ideas. The one activity I think everyone should make a part of their daily life is WALKING. My Commitment to Health was only as strong as my will to follow it through. I believe I have fulfilled it. If I could do it, so can you. Don't discount the power of activity.

Chapter 16

FACET BLOCKS

The end of October has always been an important time of the year for Sasha and me. We first met at a social function on Halloween night. A year later, on Halloween day, we married, and in 1992 we were celebrating our thirty-ninth wedding anniversary.

It was hard to believe, but for eight of our thirty-nine years of marriage I had had a health problem. Not only did I have a career carve-out; both of us had an incredible carve-out from our marital relationship. This is the impact someone can have on the lives of others through negligent operation of a motor vehicle.

This year we had planned to get away for a break, but the ongoing saga of the neck problem caused us to postpone our plans. Instead, two of our sons made a special effort, travelling considerable distances to be with us for our anniversary. They took us out for a wonderful dinner and we all had a good time. I had to rise to this occasion as for virtually every activity, but rise I did. It would have been so easy to say I was not well enough to go and everyone would have understood. It was important to me that I not carve away anything in my life that I might be able to do in spite of the difficulty. I wanted to face the daily challenges of life positively and constructively if at all possible.

After so many years of pain and problems requiring surgical intervention, you might think I was getting used to invasive medical procedures. Instead I found the opposite to be true. Each time there was a greater degree of hesitancy on my part. I was a firm believer in fixing the problem if it required fixing, but now I was also asking, "Is it going to help me? Am I being treated for the proper condition?" I had faith in the internist's diagnosis but was concerned by the speed with which it was being treated, especially given the caution and slow movement before my second fusion.

I was faced with these doubts when I went in for my first facet block. I checked in at outpatient admittance, was directed to a waiting area, and soon was called in to a sophisticated operating room where

Dr. Phil Harrison, the neuroradiologist, introduced himself to me. He told me that he would first freeze the affected area and then inject cortisone, monitoring the injection by X-ray. This week he would inject at the 2/3 level. Further injections would be at the 3/4 and 4/5 levels at two-week intervals. The two-week period between injections would allow my internist to properly assess the results.

Dr. Harrison then presented me with a release form to sign. I asked why there was a need to sign one. He explained that although he had performed this procedure many times and had never encountered a problem, there was always the possibility that one day things would go wrong, so I must give the hospital a release from liability. When I questioned him about possible problems he said that during the procedure he could hit a blood vessel or artery and this could cause a stroke. Such a scenario could leave me a quadri- or paraplegic.

His words gave me a real scare, even though I had already been exposed to the possibility of paralysis in previous surgical interventions. It must have been obvious that I was disturbed, as Dr. Harrison said that if I did not wish to go through with the procedure I could leave and think about it further.

I gave it some thought and then told him that both the internist and my personal physician had stated this was a tried and proven procedure. The request to sign a waiver form had caught me by surprise, but I understood and respected the procedure he had to follow. I went on to say that I was there for a reason and that there was not much to think about. If I was to have relief I needed to undergo this procedure. I signed the waiver form and told him I was in his hands. I had lost count of the number of waiver forms I had signed, putting myself in the hands of the medical profession – but what choice did I have?

The procedure was painful, much more than I had expected, but then how was I to know what to expect? There was an injection for the local anaesthetic and two injections of cortisone at the 2/3 level. I could picture the needles going in as I felt them, though I was not able to see the needle on the X-ray screen. I noted that the procedures were carefully done and I wondered how many more needles I would be subjected to before I was done. I had had my fill of needles by this time.

It seemed like the procedure was over in no time at all. As I walked back to the dressing room and then to our car I was very much off balance and somewhat disoriented. I felt slight relief on the drive home, but it was short-lived – I presumed it was the result of the freezing.

By the next day my neck pain was not as severe as usual when I moved my head sideways or tilted it backwards. It was a slight change, but when you are experiencing excruciating pain the slightest relief is monumental and noticeable.

Dr. Bull had asked that I come in soon after the first facet block was done. I'm sure that I looked like a person in deep distress as I sat in his office. I let him know I felt marginally less severe pain when I moved my head but added I still felt a lot of discomfort at the back of my skull. When the doctor applied some finger pressure to the area, I had a definite reaction. He told me this pain was in the trapezius muscle, which connects to the shoulder, and that he could give me some relief with an injection of cortisone. As I had to have some more facet blocks done, he recommended that I wait until they were completed.

The added stress from this new pain was not good for my blood pressure, which had shot up to 165/95. Dr. Bull decided to give me new blood pressure medication. He said I should not be too concerned as it might take a while for things to settle down. I could not help being concerned, however, as my blood pressure was going up in spite of all the relaxation techniques I practised. I realized again that no matter how much I knew about pain management, there was a threshold I could cross that always brought me to real distress. When I crossed that point my body showed it with elevated blood pressure readings. It was a vicious circle as higher blood pressure caused by stress gave me more to worry about, causing more stress.

Two weeks went by fairly quickly and I was in for another hectic day: a three-and-a-half-hour round trip to the hospital, plus the procedure of the facet block. Dr. Harrison asked me how I felt and whether there had been any change after the first injection. I told him how painful it had been for a few days and he said that this was to be expected. I also told him there had been only marginal noticeable relief, but any relief at all was much appreciated.

I was prepared for the second block, which was to be done at the 3/4 level. It was painful and the neuroradiologist apologized for hurting me, saying that he had to use a slightly different procedure. He had some difficulty getting the needle to penetrate to the correct spot. This was not too comforting for me as I immediately thought of the potential hazards I had been warned about. I gave thanks when the session was over. My immediate reaction was the same as after the first facet block and all I wanted was to get home.

By the sixth day after the second injection I felt considerable relief. There was less pain when I moved my head and I could flex my head backwards with considerably less pain. The most piercing pain was in the middle back of the skull, the same area that had been painful after the first facet block. This pain was even more pronounced and there was a considerable amount of inflammation in the area, so I began to apply ice packs at this spot.

Fourteen days after the second facet block I wrote in my diary: "I am so pleased with the progress. It is as if I am being released from a prison within my own skin. I have worked and/or done everything I could to help myself; however, if it is the facet joints and presently my improvement points to this, all I needed was the medical help to look after the problem, the rest I can manage."

I was in contact with Dr. Ong about my progress and we had to decide whether or not to do a facet block at the next level. Because I had received so much relief, she thought I should wait and see how things settled down. She had told me before the first block that this procedure was a "quick fix" and had cautioned that the most I could expect from it was some abatement of pain. There was no guarantee how long it would last.

Because of the severity of pain prior to the facet blocks, I felt it would be miraculous if I were to get any relief at all. Now it was clear that the internist had correctly diagnosed at least one of my problems and for this I was grateful to her. My philosophy of fixing the problem if it could be fixed had been proved again. More accurately, in this case we had isolated and treated the problem while realizing and accepting that the problem had not been fixed. It was a relief only, but most welcome.

Prayer and affirmations

Without going into my religious background, suffice it to say that I always repeated the Lord's Prayer to myself every night before sleep. It seemed to be the right thing to do as it was a prayer I had learned at an early age. When I was literally down and out healthwise, this was not something I had to introduce in my darkest moments. And certainly through my darkest moments there were times I literally lived on prayer. I found myself repeating the Lord's Prayer more than once a day, morning and night, yet there were times when I questioned who this prayer was directed to. "Why am I doing this?" I would ask myself, and I rationalized that if there was a hidden power I might as well take advantage of it in this time of need. It may sound strange, but I did feel a shifting of some of my worry and responsibility when I prayed.

A special prayer that I still say every morning and evening is:

I thank thee, Father, for watching over us as we rested last night.
I thank you for our family, our friends, and the populace of the
world at large.
And most of all I thank you for the God within us.
It will be a great day.
If it is going to be it is up to me. AMEN.

(In the evening I start the prayer with "I thank thee, Father, for watching over us as we rest tonight" and the penultimate line is "It was a great day.")

If a prayer is to be meaningful it must revolve around you and your circumstances. We are all different, with a host of different problems, but we all have that hot button that must be pushed over and over, even if it often seems to have no or minimal results.

After my accident I found myself dwelling on words and thoughts that were significant to me as a prisoner of my own body and pain: strength, strong, faith, trust, belief, hope, love, will, power, willpower. They came to me one at a time over a long period of my disability. They were positive and provided mental reinforcement. I found myself repeating these words over and over, all too often as a response to my medical consultations. For example, "Yes, I must have faith, trust, belief, hope in those whose care I am in." It was at times a mind game:

"Do I trust or not trust what was told me? Do I believe or not believe that I will see improvement?" Do I have faith or do I not have faith in the medical direction I am taking?"

These powerful positive power words became my affirmations and I still repeat them daily. They became part of my prayer, silent or otherwise. I believe that dwelling on these positives and prayers was helpful and healthful. At least I knew they would not destroy me as they were positive words, not negative at all.

An affirmation has to be from within oneself and must dwell on the positive. Once it is a part of you, you must repeat it so often that if there is a healing power involved, there is no doubt about its power. This power may not be noticeable on the surface, but deep within you there is no letting up on the repetition of the affirmative. In my case, because of my deteriorated health, I had to create affirmations that would reinforce my ability not only to get by on a daily basis, but also to have the necessary faith and trust in the people I was dealing with.

When I went for my walk first thing in the morning, after greeting my dog, I started to sing (and still do sing today) the following affirmation/prayer:

It is no secret what God can do
What he has done for others, he will do for you
It is no secret what he can do, what he does
for others, he'll do for you

It is no secret how much he cares
how much he cares, how much he cares
It is no secret how much he cares
how much he cares, how much he cares

It is no secret what he has done for you
what he has done for you, what he has done for you
(repeat)

It is no secret his love for you
his love for you, his love for you
(repeat)

176

It is no secret my love for him
my love for him, my love for him
(repeat)

It is no secret how much I care
how much I care, how much I care
(repeat)

It is no secret I have been forgiven
of all my sins, of all my sins
(repeat)

It is no secret that shining light
it shines on me, it shines on me
(repeat)

It is no secret you must be strong
you must be strong, you must be strong
(repeat)

It is no secret you must have strength
you must have strength, you must have strength
(repeat)

It is no secret you must have faith
you must have faith, you must have faith
(repeat)

It is no secret you must have trust
you must have trust, you must have trust
(repeat)

It is no secret you must believe
you must believe, you must believe
(repeat)

It is no secret you must have hope
you must have hope, you must have hope
(repeat)

It is no secret you must have love
you must have love, you must have love
(repeat)

It is no secret it is within me
it is within me, it is within me

It is no secret God's working with me
God's working with me, God's working with me
(repeat)

It is no secret God is within me
God is within me, God is within me
(repeat)

It is no secret you must have will
you must have will, you must have will
(repeat)

It is no secret you must have power
you must have power, you must have power
(repeat)

It is no secret you must have willpower
you must have willpower, you must have willpower
(repeat)

It is no secret I will overcome
I will overcome, I will overcome
(repeat)

It is no secret, it's in my hands
it's in my hands, it's in my hands
(repeat)

It is no secret, I am in his hands
I am in his hands, I am in his hands
(repeat)

It is no secret, if it's going to be
it's up to me, it's up to me
(repeat)

I sang this every day as it reminded me of what belief in God can do. What he has done for others, he would also do for me. God's work is well known and when you let him inside you, in his own way he will heal. Give him the work to do and let the power of the unspoken word, the power from above, silently, though not necessarily knowingly, heal.

The first affirmations reminded me that God cares and the caring is everlasting. The problem for us is to let God in and to show that we too care. We must not open our heart occasionally but must allow him to share in all of our victories as well as adversities. When we are troubled it can be particularly difficult to see what he has done for us and to wait for our prayers to be answered, but we must not stop asking for help. We may not get a direct answer, but there will be some response. If you have never opened your heart to God, it may not be easy at first. If you are troubled, you can speak to him silently and he will hear you.

I reminded myself of my love for him, so deep and true, so private and unashamed. I care for him and for what he does. It may not be visible, but what matters is inside. For many years I have lived with a vision of radiating white light shining on me. I first saw it early one morning as I was out for my walk. As I prayed, I felt rays of light that not only shone on me but were penetrating. It was as if I had a new-found power and I believed then, and still do, that it was an answer to my prayers. This vision is so powerful that I can literally bring it on at any time. In moments of difficulty it is a powerful, uplifting force.

I also remembered that if I ask for forgiveness, I shall receive it. Though I feel I have lived a relatively sinless life, there is not a day goes by when I don't do something that requires forgiveness. I have always lived with forgiveness in mind and feel each and every day should end with forgiveness.

"It is no secret you must be strong." Having been through so much trauma, I liken myself to a brick wall. It did not matter which way I turned, I was trapped and there was no way out. I had to be strong from within with all my medical advisors and with all of those people I had contact with on a daily basis. I had to have nerves of steel to meet the challenge of each and every day and feel good about it.

As well as strength I needed faith – faith in myself and faith in those who were entrusted with my health. I lived and breathed faith so strongly that at times this was all the strength I could come up with when there were hair-raising decisions being made about my life. I had to have trust, trust that was beyond belief when I was putting my life in someone else's hands. I lost count of how many times this happened, but I had an unfailing trust. I had to believe in myself and in others, particularly my surgeons. One slip of a scalpel and heaven knows where I could have ended up. I shall be forever grateful I was in such skilled hands.

Hope was another important element. Hope is a difficult concept to describe as I do not believe you live and survive on hope. Hope is nebulous, yet very real. It is the wanting and craving of something special – for me it was the hope of ever-improving health each and every day.

"It is no secret you must have love." There is no question that my love reached out to all of those who cared for me through my difficult times - God, self, spouse, family, and the world at large. To love those around you can at times be difficult, but those transgressors must answer for themselves.

It was no secret that my problem was within me, but God was working with me and I literally put my problems in God's hands. I felt then, as I do now, when that shining light shone on me I was in God's hands.

While you believe that the Divine Power is watching over you and helping you, you also must have the will, willpower, and determination to stay on track, especially when suffering from distress. You must maintain total control over your positive thoughts and not allow the negative to rule you. It is so easy to fall into a trap where you lose all your willpower to fight, to carry on. You question "What's the use?" However, if you transform all of those negative forces into positive willpower, the challenge is on. Every negative thought must, through willpower, be replaced with a positive one. Power from within propels you. Over my many years of adversity, there were prolonged periods in which I could barely muster up my power, yet with prayer and the help of God I was able to sustain myself from day to day.

When I was down and out, one of the most difficult things was to keep feeding myself positive affirmations when all looked like doom and gloom. However, this was where I felt I must continually rise to the occasion and overrule negative thoughts with positive ones. It required a lot of repetition, but I kept at it.

Remember "If it's going to be, it is up to me." When you are ill, a big part of recovery lies with the individual. Medical help plays a part, but I tried to put the responsibility of getting better squarely on my own shoulders, with no one to answer to but myself. I sought medical care and then resolved that the rest was up to me. Just knowing that I was carrying my share of the load gave me a high degree of satisfaction.

This was the significance of the lyrics that I sang every day. As I sang, I mindfully explored the meanings of the words. On different days there was more emphasis on some verses than on others. They had special meaning depending on my needs that day. I did not rush through my lyrics, as I wanted to get something positive from them each and every day.

Dwelling on positives and prayers is more healthy than brooding about negative thoughts. I know that I still use them daily, and I firmly believe that anyone who uses prayer and affirmation daily will at least have more inner peace. The healing powers will look after themselves.

You can make up your own prayers and affirmations. You do not need a large vocabulary of positive words to work with. What you need are words to match your problem at a given time, and this could require some research. What is important is to have prayers that are special to you, with meaning to you. My affirmations and choice of words could be a launching pad for your own lyric. Add, delete, use them as they are, but get started now.

There is another positive message I refer to often. A number of years ago while scavenging in an antique store, I came across a plaque that was of immediate interest to me. The message gave me the strangest feeling, as if it had been written yesterday. It is "Desiderata" by Max Ehrmann, the prayer/meditation that begins "Go placidly amid the noise and haste, and remember what peace there may be in silence."

I brought the plaque home and cleaned it up, and now it occupies a prominent spot between our kitchen and dining room. I have read this plaque every day for years. In my most troubled times I would read it a number of times a day. I found the writing so inspirational that I believe it helped carry me through some troubled times.

Don't discount the power of prayer and affirmations. I *can* state that the use of affirmations and prayer helped me. And if this God to whom we pray did in fact answer my prayers, I will be forever grateful.

Chapter 17

ANOTHER NEW YEAR

I was now entering the ninth year of fighting my burden of pain and I was as determined as ever to beat it. When I was healthy I always felt I had complete control of any situation; now an unknown force had a grip on me and I was virtually helpless to do anything but cope from day to day. No matter how tough I thought I was and how capable of withstanding the unknown, this was one unknown I wished I had never encountered.

After the facet block I started to experience some relief from the pain. It was like a yo-yo, up and down, whereas before the facet block the pain had been a vise-grip twenty-four hours a day. I was always praying for a good day, though the facet block was certainly not a quick fix. It gave me an inch and I would take a mile, constantly testing myself. Often I would overdo an activity and face the consequences. I had gained more mobility in my head, but not without an all-enveloping skull pain, and I continued to have problems when sitting, standing, walking, bending forward from a standing position, writing, driving. This pain would intensify as the day wore on, and the area was tender to the touch with continued inflammation.

Dr. Bull told me the problem was the trapezius muscle and tendon and said he would give me a cortisone injection after my next visit to the internist. The trapezius is a large, powerful, diamond-shaped muscle between the neck and the shoulders. It helps to hold the shoulder blade in position and rotates it and also helps to rotate the head on the trunk – or hold the neck and skull still. I was protecting myself as much as possible from head movements that come naturally when one is well, and this effort was causing the muscle to go into spasm and become inflamed. Cortisone would ease the inflammation and thus lessen the pain.

The skull rotates at the 2/3 level facet joint – a delicate area (frankly I do not know of an area in our body that is not delicate) – so was it any wonder I was having problems? The human body was not built to withstand the forces that can crunch metal.

When I drove or rode in a car I no longer felt the severe compounded pain when the vehicle stopped or started. This alone was a big improvement. Not total relief, but enough that I did not have to be vocal, crying out at the instant pain. In late January 1993 we decided to visit one of our daughters and her family in Campbell River. The trip to their home, including a ferry ride, was a six-hour journey. We stayed three days and, quite frankly, I was in so much pain that I wanted to turn around and go right home as soon as we arrived. I needed to rest and have things settle down. I used to thrive on going out for a drive and thought nothing of it before my injury. Now a trip like this was too much for me.

At the end of the month Sasha and I went dining and dancing. We had a lovely evening, but not without a price for me. It had become our way of life. I was damned if I did and damned if I didn't, so I would choose the road of damned if I did. There was a flip side to the coin and that was that both of us enjoyed an intimate evening. Life goes on, life is for living, and we have to learn how to mix the good with the bad no matter how difficult it may be.

I was spending some time each day cleaning out my office files. This was a positive activity for me because in the previous four years I had not touched this material. There were many times I had wanted to start unpacking but had been unable to because I had such a low level of concentration due to the amount of medication I was taking.

I continued to be so anxious to get well that with every bit of relief I would start to test myself gradually, only to find regression setting in every time. As an example, shortly after undergoing the facet blocks I thought I would try my rowing machine, which had not been used for many years. I started out with a few pulls a day and after four days I could feel things starting to change – for the worse. I immediately stopped the activity. In my diary I wrote: "It takes a man of steel to continue to have hope and faith when facing such adversities and to keep yourself going from day to day, restraining yourself to within your limitations."

After the facet block I was able to slowly cut back on the medication I was taking. Over the years I had learned how to self-

184

medicate. I would be given a prescription with a recommended dosage. Though I was not one to take a lot of pills, by prescription or otherwise, because of my condition I needed them to give me relief from pain. If I found the medication was helping I would cut back on the dosage to where I was tolerating pain within my limitations. If I cut back too much I soon knew it and would increase the dosage to a level where it kept me at a subdued level of pain. Nothing I was taking was going to heal me; the pills were simply there to give relief, so my philosophy was "Why take more than I have to?" If it did not help whatsoever, I would stop taking it and try something else. I took only the medication that gave me some relief and took only the amount needed to help me from day to day.

I used a variety of methods to fight the excruciating pain: ice packs, hot packs, rest and relaxation (how much more rest do I need? I often wondered), meditation, self-hypnosis, audio and video tapes – you name it, I tried it. Any one of the many procedures probably helped keep me from deteriorating further at that time. I was trying to reach a plateau, a lower level of pain, and I would try any method that might help me gain relief. The facet blocks showed that all that medication and all the pain-management techniques were band-aids. The real solution was to get a shot of cortisone into the root of the problem. I continued to have pain, but I was taking much less medication and on the odd day, none at all.

In mid-February 1993 I entered the following in my diary: "Overall I am extremely pleased with my progress since the facet blocks. I can actually feel myself getting better, stronger, with the ability to last the day and not in total pain. To this day, I consider the facet blocks nothing short of a miracle, one day I was in a total disaster situation and then relieved of the debilitating pain which had haunted me since the July 1991 accident. A long time to be kept in suspense as to my health and whether or not, when it came to the crunch, the facet blocks would be helpful. What a relief and now, hopefully, the trapezius can be looked after, the rest is all inside me and there is nothing I can do here except accept that there is a long term deteriorating situation and that hopefully I will be able to at least function without being in total pain on a day-to-day basis."

After writing these positive observations, my next day's activity shows how I was constantly testing the waters. Some close friends spoke often of how much they enjoyed their involvement in a five-pin bowling league. I always envied any of my friends when they spoke of their various physical activities and had come to accept that I could not participate in my present condition. However, these stories of bowling hit a nerve. I used to bowl in a men's commercial league and my blood was boiling to give bowling a try, so Sasha and I arranged to go bowling with another couple.

By the seventh frame of the first game I was in a lot of pain and wondered if I was going to make it to the tenth frame and the end of the game. I did my best to conceal the compounded pain I was in and not only made it to the last frame but also continued to play two more games as we'd planned. I was out to test myself and I paid the price, but I rationalized that I was again facing a "Damned if you do and damned if you don't" choice. If I wanted to have some enjoyment, I knew there had to be a trade-off, but the trade of enjoyment for compounded pain did not seem a fair one.

In the latter part of February I had an appointment with Dr. Ong. Although I was not without ongoing problems, she noted significant change in the way I was carrying myself compared to before the facet blocks. She was pleased to see me smiling and to see the increased mobility I had in my head. She said that with proper management the facet blocks could carry me for a long time and that I was welcome to see her at any time.

I expressed my gratitude for what she had done for me and asked what she thought of my going away for a vacation. She gave me her blessing, as had my personal physician, and suggested I try to do some swimming as the exercise would be good for me.

It seemed strange to be going on a vacation when I was normally confined to my home surroundings, but both my wife and I had earned it and for Sasha it was long overdue. The philosophy of "Give me an inch of health and I will take a mile" prevailed.

At the end of February, one of our sons drove us to a hotel in Richmond, near the Vancouver airport, where we stayed overnight for our early flight to Ixtapa the next morning. This was our third trip to

Mexico and on the flight I savoured my many pleasant memories of Mexico, its fine people, its culture, and especially the weather.

On our first day in Ixtapa I could not resist the warm water of the hotel pool. After being in the water for a while, temptation got the best of me and I did the sidestroke, as suggested by the internist. It only took the width of the pool, there and back, to find out where I was. It was not good. I had severe compounded pain radiating from my neck and shoulder area to the skull at pre-facet block levels of pain. I could not believe it and thought it might be something else. However, as I sat in a deck chair I said to myself, "Don't panic and see the house doctor. This is just a repeat performance."

The pain was so severe that it was hard to accept it was the same old thing, but by the next day, when there was no let up, I knew it was true. I was back on medication and, in my mind, ready to go home. Only two days here and all the joy had been taken away by a few sidestrokes in a pool of water. "How ridiculous," I thought as I realized I should have known better. But then I reasoned, how would I know if I did not try?

It took nine days before things settled down. That took a lot of the fun out of the vacation. After all, I thought, I could have easily discovered this when I was at home. But then I turned it around again. Had I gone for a discovery swim at home and found out what condition I was in, we would probably not be in Ixtapa. That was the end of the self-blaming.

The most difficult part of the trip for me was the travel to and from airports. No matter how much I tried to brace myself, it was impossible to prevent the forward and backward sway with every start and stop of the vehicle. And with every sway I felt compounded neck pain radiating up the back of the skull. I just had to grin and bear it. What else could I do?

In my diary after returning home I wrote: "The swimming attempt did not prove to be favourable and I am scratching any of this type of activity in the future. I have been burned too many times and it is absolutely ludicrous to hurt yourself knowingly. Yet how do you know where you are at until you try? I continue to tolerate a level of pain which is tolerable, yet even this level of pain would be intense if it were not for learning how to cope."

187

I had scheduled an appointment with Dr. Bull after our return home and instead of presenting myself relaxed and rested, I was a wreck. He was most sympathetic and decided to give me a cortisone injection in the area of the trapezius muscle, as the back of my skull continued to be bothersome and painful.

Two days after the injection into the trapezius muscle I wrote: "In light of the most recent problems I have had, the facet joints and now the trapezius being attended to, I know that I personally could not do anything more for myself other than endure the torture that went with it. Amen!!"

On the negative side, on March 18 I wrote: "It is such a tight, firm, deep clenching pain that I have learned to cope with that an ordinary human being, not having experienced anything like it, would be putting in an emergency call to their doctor."

And so it went. I continued to tolerate the pain and cope, often wondering if it was a new problem, if it was possible for any pain to last this long, if I should take more medication and tolerate less pain? Pain management is a full-time job, twenty-four hours a day, and real pain is difficult to live with no matter how much one learns about pain management. It is a force beyond compare.

I received a little relief from the injection into the trapezius muscle, though not as much as I had expected. Perhaps I always expected too much. It was six weeks before I had some relief after the attempt at swimming in Ixtapa. My personal physician noted that should I have further regression, it might be advisable to have further facet blocks. I cringed at the thought of another invasive treatment. Even though I had come through so many procedures without any problems, I had heard too much about the chance of becoming paralyzed as a result of these treatments. If I felt any fear it was of becoming a quadri- or paraplegic. The thought of having to sign yet another form releasing the surgeon and hospital from liability should I be crippled was scary.

On April 16 I wrote: "It is unfortunate that I continue to find myself in such a delicate situation. I do not have to do anything!!! just sit in a theatre for a few hours!!! how and when will this ever end?? and is this the way it is going to be forever? If so, I have a lot of difficulty in accepting the fact that there is nothing more which can be done. I refuse to accept the word disabled, yet in reality I am not only disabled, but must pay a high price on a daily basis for virtually any type of activity/inactivity which I partake in. It is a living hell, yet I am grateful for what health I have and will continue to make the most of each and every day."

I finished the entry on a positive note. "Will continue to make the most of each and every day." By putting it in writing as often as I did, I reinforced my commitment to do all I could to get back to better health. Putting my problems down in pen and ink also served to give me a sense of perspective. The written word is powerful medicine.

Ten days later I wrote: "On the positive side, this is what has been happening. A settling effect, not without pain, however, incredibly improved over the constant excruciating pain prior to the facet blocks. I am having better days. I only hope and pray that they will turn into yet considerably better days.

"Frankly, it is very discouraging, yet I must stay positive despite the ongoing frustrations. I must look back and compare where I was and where I am today."

Again, this was positive self-reinforcement. By writing out my thoughts I could better reflect on them and could also see a gradual improvement. I could not measure my progress in days, weeks, or even months. All too often there was absolutely no progress – and at times there was regression instead – in my condition. However, when I looked at the big picture over half a year, a year, two years, or back to my original state, I could see that I had made tremendous progress. It was this type of positive thinking that I found was necessary to focus on daily and even hourly on many occasions.

At the end of April my notes read: "In any event, the plateau I am at presently is a milestone compared to six months ago, pre the facet block period. If only I could now get total relief. It matters not what I do, literally nothing, just carrying the head – hard to believe but again experience has shown me that there is obviously aggravation on a day to day basis. I will continue to push myself. I will endure. What choice do I have? At the very least, if I have ultimate near full recovery, it will have been because I refused to give up.

"The no pain, no gain syndrome may not necessarily apply. However, with pain, I have proven that you can do something each and every day over a long period of time. The fruits of your labours do show. I have been functioning at a new found speed and if I was being paid for what I do, however menial, I would have been fired a long time ago."

I was starting to feel better; not without pain but feeling stronger on a daily basis with highs and lows. The highs were simply a better day. The lows were the bottom of the barrel.

In early May I made the following notes in my diary: "As soon as I have a good day, my mind goes a mile a minute on all the things I want to do, yet I know I have to be careful as I can set myself back in a minute."

By mid-May I noted: "I do wonder how I ever tolerated and lived through the past. I must continue my quest for better health. It is just that it has me baffled as to what, if anything, I could do now to get better yesterday. Why do they not have the answers to my problem? Maybe they do have the answers and are not able to help a condition such as mine any more than what has been done."

It was obvious that time was necessary for healing and there were no quick fixes. A positive development was that my blood pressure was back to normal so I was able to stop taking one set of pills. The stress, the strain, and the severe pain had moderated and so had the blood pressure. I continued to use all the self-help techniques for pain management on a daily basis and I started to find that after a session of self-help the pain levels would moderate somewhat, unlike in the past when I seldom noticed any significant difference before and after a session.

Something as simple as a game of pool was a measure of my progress. We have a billiard table in our home and as well as enjoying a game of pool with whoever wanted to play, I would rack up the balls and clear the table on my own. Immediately after my accident I could not bend over the table and hold my head upwards to aim my cue. I had to learn to use the cue from a totally upright standing position. By May 1993 I was starting to flex my head backwards – not without pain, but the ability to bend over and to hold my head backwards was definite progress.

By late May I was mowing the lawn and recorded that I was not having as much difficulty with this activity. I had marked improvement in head movement and was suffering substantially reduced pain levels from a year before. This was another advantage of keeping a diary. I would not have remembered time frames so well without it, and being able to look back and see how far I had progressed was a positive reinforcement.

Reading was less difficult and I noticed that my concentration and retention levels had vastly improved. I was even taking an interest in technical material pertinent to my career. It was a long time coming, but I was starting to see a little glimmer at the other end of the tunnel. It was as if I were climbing a mountain that became higher as I climbed. I was determined to reach the top.

By mid-June, however, I felt I was regressing. It did not happen overnight but crept up slowly. I realized the pain was increasing and I was in more pain earlier each day. As I reflected on my activities of the previous weeks I was able to see that I had been feeling better, I had become more active, and though I thought I was careful, I had been doing more than I was capable of.

Healing is a constant learning process. You always have to be alert to what you are doing, what you have done, what you are going to do...must always be guarded because you do not want to set yourself back. Self-diagnosis, self-control, self-critique, self-medication, self-management, self, self, self.

In the third week of June I had another injection of cortisone in the back of the skull. It was easy for Dr. Bull to pinpoint the troubled area as it was inflamed and tender to the touch. Although I was still in pain, it was not excruciating and my blood pressure readings were back to normal without the need of medication. This was most positive, as I had seen my blood pressure soar in the past when I was totally stressed out from pain.

At this visit we also discussed the further regression in the neck area. The doctor told me this was probably due to the fact that the cortisone was wearing off. I had to decide whether I would have further facet blocks or let the body heal on its own.

I am not one to procrastinate, but I was procrastinating about having more facet blocks as I had a great fear of being left in worse shape. I had a bellyfull of pain-management techniques and while they had not seemed to make any difference in the past, now there were positive results when I used them. I was feeling some relief, and the fact that I was having the occasional better day convinced me that I should continue to tolerate the pain on my own and see what happened.

On July 1 I noted in my diary: "Then there is the activity and/or no activity syndrome. Just sitting brings on pain. It is hard to believe that here I am with yet another half a year gone. I have never experienced time as I have during my illness. Days running into weeks, weeks running into months, months running into years. An interruption in our lifestyle beyond compare, a shattering career interruption not to mention the monetary loss. Fortunately, I have been able to cope, however, it gnaws at me on a daily basis and this prolonged interruption is extremely frustrating.

"The move to the country, particularly this piece of property, has been very therapeutic in that I have created some interesting projects. However, my heart is in my career and as I reflect on my progress, perhaps the fact that I live from day to day in the hope that I am going to work, this in itself has probably played a major role in my recovery, if in fact I can call it recovery at this stage. Without question I am a lot better than I was during the pre-facet block period which in itself is gratifying."

On July 8 I wrote: "As I write these notes at eight-thirty a.m., the neck area is enveloped in pain. It is difficult to cope and understand the why of the continued aggravation. Perhaps another way of putting it is, with all the advanced technology it is difficult to comprehend why there is not a quick fix so you can get well and get on with life as you used to know it. Fortunately, I am at the very least able to look after myself. I am forever grateful for having the strength to be able to carry on in the hope that this will all be behind me in due time. The due time is long overdue."

At times I found I was questioning the positive thinking I fed myself as it was in direct conflict with what was actually happening with my health. Nevertheless, the mind over matter effort of staying positive kept me from being swallowed up by the negatives.

And I was dealing with a lot of negatives. In spite of the present slow recovery, the whole experience was negative because it was so prolonged. I continued to have faith that with time I would get better. There had been many days when it seemed like that time would never come, but now I was starting to see glimmers of light. I was starting to have the occasional better day. When you have been down and out for years, this is a revelation. One day of feeling better and I was elated. The next day, down and out again, I was deflated. Though I was thrilled to have good days, this variability required adjustment as it was not what I had been used to.

With the slightest improvement I was testing myself to the limit. I wasn't going to an extreme of activity. I was just pushing that little bit more and I was not ready for it. It could be that I would have regressed even if I had not exerted myself. The healing process moves up and down.

Pain management had become a way of life. On July 12 I wrote: "I continue my rest periods, meditation, self-hypnosis, walking, self-talk, affirmations, prayer...you name it, I do it! I believe I have tried and continue to do everything positive in my recovery and recover I will.

"I have not and do not dwell on the negatives. Surely with my very difficult days it would have been easy to go with the flow. However, I accepted there was something wrong and in my own way fought and continue to fight."

Even though there were ups and downs from day to day, I found that my inner strength was increasing. I had many affirmations that I repeated on a daily basis and my self-talk and beliefs brightened the other end of the tunnel, which had been dark for many years. I wrote: "I now also see shimmers of light which give me, and reinforce, the sustaining strength which somehow I have been able to hold on to."

In late July I had a telephone call from Lawrence, a former colleague whom I had known for many years. Over ten years earlier Lawrence had told me he needed to have surgery on a blocked carotid artery. When we originally discussed it, and on subsequent occasions, he agonized over his situation, the life-threatening nature of the surgery, and his reluctance to undergo the operation while his daughter was still a child. He also recognized the life-threatening nature of the blocked artery, which could kill him at any time, but he hoped to live at least long enough to see his daughter grow up.

It was a heavy load to carry. I vividly recall discussing with Lawrence the decision he had to make and telling him that if I were in his position, I believed I would opt for the surgery: "You know you have a problem, you are concerned about it, it is constantly on your mind – you should get it fixed and get on with life." It was easy to say, but I was saying it to the person who required the surgery and those were not his sentiments. His fear – "What if I don't make it?" – kept coming through loud and clear.

I had to agree that his daughter needed him, but "What if it gets worse?" I would ask him.

His response was, "I would go quickly."

Lawrence called me now to tell me that he had recovered from major surgery. The artery had been 95 percent blocked, but the surgery had been successful and the surgeon told Lawrence, "You will never have to see me again." He was elated and apologized for not letting me know in advance, but he felt I had enough on my plate as it was.

He went on to say that it was as if he had been let out of prison. I told him that I felt the same way. I was still a prisoner but with daily freedom passes to do whatever I wished, and I felt I was a model prisoner because I did not have to have a monitor attached to me.

In late July my personal physician again changed my anti-inflammatory medication. Any medication taken over a prolonged period of time may lose some of its effectiveness. This had happened with the drug I was taking and I was pleased to find the new medication gave me some relief. We also discussed further facet blocks, but agreed to stick with our wait-and-see approach.

At the end of July an excerpt from my notes reads: "The tolerance for pain and managing it is incredible. The pain has been enough to drive me to drugs, alcohol or whatever. You must have strength, be strong and have faith and belief that you will overcome. I pray that one day I will be drug free of prescription drugs. I continue to find it difficult to accept and/or believe that I have a medical problem that cannot be fixed."

In mid-August my diary reads: "Without question, I have just had two of the best days back to back since the July 1991 accident. I could start jumping for joy. However, I am still on medication and do have shoulder, neck radiating to skull pain. But the tremendous settling effect over the last two days is welcome relief. In fact, what I am tolerating would in the normal scheme of things be intolerable by the average person who has never been subjected to such trauma. I will take what I can get, and only hope for yet better days."

One day later my diary reads: "Today I went to town with one of my sons and although he is a very careful driver, he descended our country road at what would be normal speeds for drivers on our road, certainly much faster than I do, which is in first gear all the time. With the accelerated speed, the braking and the curves in the road, the pain radiating to the skull was quite severe. I knew I was not out of the woods. What was very positive was that by the end of the day the pain levels had settled. This was unlike the past where I would at times go for days before there was any settling whatsoever.

"As I return from my daily walks, rather than being in severe compounded skull pain it is very much moderated."

Without a doubt the medication was holding me together. After the episode of riding in a vehicle with my son, my notes read: "The setback I have suffered since July 1991 has and continues to tax me to limits which I did not know I had and hope I can sustain these strengths."

When I suddenly suffered severe skull pain after a couple of good days, I could not help but wonder how much longer I would have to put up with this type of health. I was finding that being on a rollercoaster presented a new set of problems. When I was in constant pain, positive thought processes had become integrated into my daily life. With the highs and the lows I was now experiencing, the positive thought processes were continually being interrupted. I had to adapt to yet another change in this healing process.

In some ways it was frustrating. I would enjoy better days and then the downside would seem worse than ever. I could not help but wonder which was real, the upside or the downside, but I stayed positive and took the downside as part of the healing process, always in the hope that I was guessing right.

I also had to adapt my daily activities. In the past it was "Slow as a turtle but steady wins the race"; now I was finding myself in a stop-and-go predicament. In the past, if I overexerted myself I would know immediately or within a day or two. All I had to do was think about what I had done in the previous few days and I could pinpoint the source of the additional setback.

With the ups and downs, a new type of reality set in. In late August I wrote: "It is a difficult period. I have had days where there seems to be a light at the end of the tunnel. Then there are fair days and then days like yesterday. Over the years I have been able to handle problems of virtually any kind which faced me, both personal and business. Mind over matter. However, this matter is a killer. It has me in a vise grip and there is no way out. Is there further disk deterioration? Is there a nerve being pinched? I have gone through so much with this latest episode and see little progress. Major in that I do have neck mobility since the facet blocks and initially a lot of relief from pain, however, there has been a slow, subtle transformation taking place and I know I have regressed. Is it only the facet joints? Is it something else? Am I going to be burdened with this condition the rest of my life? Will it get worse? Pain management is one thing, pain management with medication is another. It is downright disgusting."

I got rid of everything bothering me on paper and got on with my life as best I could. My rationale was that I had come this far; even if the continuing pain was beyond my comprehension, I was out to beat it at all odds. And although I was continuing to go through some difficult times, I could not help but think that with a mixture of fair and better days, a change was coming about. I felt I was settling into a new plateau in my recovery.

In early September my diary notes that one of my sons was out for the weekend to get some pre-cut dried wood in for the winter. I helped with the stacking and wrote: "If I look at the big picture, a year, my condition has improved markedly. I could definitely feel additional pain from the wood piling exercise, another damned if you do and damned if you don't situation. A positive sign is that additional pain created from the activity or no activity has settled overnight. Unlike in the past where the pain was so strong that activity or no activity there was no recognizing various pain levels. I am most pleased, but completely baffled as to the various pain levels. For example, additional pain levels yesterday, quite strong by late afternoon, settled by this morning. I shall look upon this as a positive aggravation, settling in a much shorter period of time."

Another noticeable positive was that my pain-management techniques were having results. Instead of having equal levels of pain before and after a session, I was now feeling some relief and was beginning to believe that what I had been doing was beneficial to me even when there had been no noticeable relief.

I wrote: "It is both incredible and wonderful if I may use the word wonderful for a setback. In the past it was pain twenty-four hours a day, intense. Now, although there is pain, it is subdued compared to the past, however, more importantly, when aggravated, there is a settling effect by the next day. A big change is taking place and I hope and pray that it is indeed the light at the other end of the tunnel."

Feeling somewhat better, I had an office framed in an area of our house that originally was partitioned to be a nanny's room. The area was still unfinished when we bought the home and I had immediately earmarked it for an office. Now it had everything I would need to get myself operating as a life insurance agent out of my home. Filing files and shelving boxes of books took many days. I had learned to pace myself, slow but sure.

As we moved into fall I discussed with Sasha my desire to try an outside activity for the winter months. I was feeling better and felt I needed to test myself, so I joined a five-pin bowling league for men and women aged fifty-five and up. It was an early afternoon league and I felt this would give me a good part of the day after bowling to rest and recover.

By the fifth frame in the first game I was in total pain, which remained for the rest of the afternoon. Most readers will know the basics of how bowling works: players roll a ball down a lane to knock down five bowling pins. A game is made up of ten frames or turns. In each frame a player gets three chances to knock all the pins down. If you knock them all down on your first shot it's called a "strike" and you don't need to use your other two tries. So by the fifth frame I could have been putting strain on my neck, shoulder, and skull anywhere from five to fifteen times, depending on how accurate my shots were. And I could feel this strain. The neck/skull pain was absolute punishment - literally self-inflicted punishment as it was obviously the result of my bowling. After not having bowled for over ten years, my scores for the three games that first afternoon were 130, 187, and 170. (To put this in perspective, when I bowled in the 1950s my average score was 190.) I took the game seriously and was competitive, but I was also protecting myself from pain, not playing as loosely as I would have before my injury. Nonetheless, I did enjoy the game and was pleased that I was able to tolerate the pain as well as I did.

I was in a lot of discomfort for the rest of the day, but by the next morning the pain levels had settled to the status quo. My diary reads: "This in itself is remarkable. Before, it was intense pain twenty-four hours a day, only to be further compounded by any type of activity. I note that given the least bit of relief the old saying of give me an inch and I'll take a mile applies. I have continually reached and/or stretched to my limits and when you are striving for better health, it can be very difficult and especially so when you see those around you enjoying all of the amenities of life which are of interest to them."

In early September I recorded: "Visited mother today. Drove there and back by myself. Overall I had a fair trip. Generally, by the time I get home from a trip like this I have been wiped out for the day with compounded pain. On this trip, when I got home, although not without some shoulder/neck pain, I felt good enough to spend some time cutting the lawn. This, plus a drive to town, back to back to yesterday's bowling and not in extreme pain is a big turn around. If the ups and downs I have been having are and were a sign of getting better, I believe it is for real. Nevertheless, I will not start doing cartwheels yet, probably never will, however, it is great to be feeling better, noticeably so."

My journal was starting to have some exciting and positive entries, which had an even greater therapeutic effect. I was feeling good, writing how I felt. There was a lingering question – "Is this really true? Is this really happening to me?" But since it was my philosophy to say it (or write it) the way I saw it, I knew it was true. I truly was feeling better.

In mid-September Sasha and I made a car trip to visit one of our sons. For me this two-and-a-half-hour shared drive was yet another test of my condition. "Overall I had a fair trip. As I write these notes, I am with shoulder, neck pain, however, there is no comparison as to our last trip there earlier this year. I have had quite a number of fair days, back to back and with what I would call a fair amount of activity – very promising – I am elated!!!! – it is an incredible feeling to have *so much relief*!"

A few days after the trip I noted: "I have been for my walk and although in some pain, not intense, settled over night. If I am settling into another plateau it is like night and day to what I have been used to. In the past, predictable in that the pain was with me twenty-four hours a day. Now it is incredibly unpredictable. This is not to say I would predict pain, it was that I was enveloped in total pain and it mattered not what I did. At the very most, in the latter stages some relief. I will take this as a plateau and reach for the next one."

By late September the bowling was taking its toll. "As I reflect on the last few weeks, I am slowly regressing. I can only assume that I am hurting myself and the trade off is not pleasant. I have had more than enough stress, pain and suffering.

"However, unless I continue to test myself how will I know where I am at? In a sense it continues to be a damned if you do situation. The stressful pain and suffering is now self-inflicted and I do not realize how much I have hurt myself until after the fact.

"I believe we are all prisoners of our own bodies from the day we are born. However, when you have a medical condition such as I have, no matter what I try to do there is a force stronger than I am."

In early October my journal says: "What is incredible is, when I look at the big picture, a year or two ago a trip to town and back, twenty-one miles, was an ordeal and on many occasions I had no choice but to be a passenger in a vehicle. Things were looking up, although I find it hard to comprehend the rollercoaster up and down condition I am having. However, I believe it is the beginning of the light at the other end of the tunnel, even though it fades out quite often. It takes a lot of willpower to continue maintaining various activities when I have negative results."

During my years of disability I made sure that we got out to the theatre and the occasional symphony performance. It was an ordeal and a pleasure each time, though the ordeal far overruled and detracted from the pleasure. The most difficult part of any performance was to sit through it with the constant neck pain radiating to the skull. After attending a live theatre performance in mid-October, I wrote: "The most significant part of the evening was that by the end of the evening I was not in excruciating pain as I have been in the past after sitting with no support for a number of hours."

What a welcome relief it was to be able to go to the theatre and enjoy it. I knew that with this let-up from severe pain I was into another plateau. Not out of the woods, but what a revelation. I had been having better days, but not to this degree. It was as if my body said, "Here, try this and see how you like it." If that was what it was doing, I liked it!

My bowling continued to be a harrowing experience, but once I have started something it takes an awful lot to give it up. Furthermore, I looked upon bowling as a form of physiotherapy, stretching myself within my capabilities, deliberately punishing myself, using the "No pain, no gain" philosophy. I knew by now that my body was not healed, but I also felt that I would persevere as long as I could.

Bowling in these early months proved to be an experience of another sort as well. It seems to me that when you are overwhelmed with pain, you suffer a form of distraction, a degree of absent-mindedness or forgetfulness. I had made some errors and though one of the staff people at the bowling alley told me I was priceless, I was concerned lest these were signs of a developing pattern rather than honest errors in the course of a day.

It takes some time to adjust to a new environment. This was especially tricky at the bowling alley, a two-story building, because we bowled on alternate floors from week to week. My first error was when I went to wet my towel, walking through a set of open doors to the washroom. As I walked out it seemed like the whole bowling alley knew I was in there. I had only been in the room for a matter of seconds and fortunately there were no women in there. I was reminded it was a LADIES washroom, not LADDIES.

On another occasion, Sasha asked me if I had my shoes when I returned home from bowling. Certainly I have my shoes, I responded. Then she asked me if I had my own shoes, as someone from the bowling alley had called inquiring as to whether I had changed into a wrong pair of shoes. I was adamant my shoes were my own, but when we checked them it turned out they were indeed someone else's shoes. Same style of shoe, same colour, same size. It was embarrassing, but I chalked it up to an honest mistake. After all, why did someone leave the same style of shoes next to mine?

Another time, after I had said good day to the staff member and was on my way out, she called me back because I had forgotten to take my bowling shoes with me.

Because I had been a perfectionist all my life, these errors were out of the ordinary. What seemed funny to others was downright embarrassing for me. However, I took the attitude that life goes on and these mistakes meant that I quickly became known to everyone at the bowling alley in a strange sort of way.

Around this time I attempted to cut back on the medication, but my body was not ready for this. Because the medication was helping to hold me together, my doctor and I decided to stay with it rather than use further invasive facet blocks.

On October 17 I wrote: "For me as a lay person and having lived with a problem for a prolonged period of time, I can only come to the conclusion that I am positively on the mend."

Then on October 21: "It is a beautiful time of the year and for this I am grateful, especially here where we see so much of nature. This morning the geese flying overhead, honking away. I picked some walnuts the other day and left them on our verandah to dry, however, the Steller's jay is picking them up at the rate of one or two a day. Our friend the bear in the apple tree must have hit the ground quite hard the other day as he came down, breaking a fairly big branch. The deer are in the yard daily. Unbelievable but true, I am still picking raspberries daily while a grouse flutters through the scrub. When we go for our walk, Duchess loves it when a rabbit shows up – they outsmart her every time.

"Without a doubt it has been therapeutic living here, difficult, but peaceful, so close to nature as an eagle soars over head."

My ups and downs continued to be recorded in my diary. In late October I wrote: "It is very disheartening, yet if I stop and reflect, I have come a long way. I do not have as severe radiating pain to the skull with head movement. The radiating pain to the skull with stops and starts of a vehicle while driving and as a passenger has markedly subsided. Presently I have considerably less skull pain when I move my head backwards. Definitely a lot of progress, but it is so slow for a workaholic and with improvement, if that is what it is, it is even more difficult to keep the brakes on. There is no doubt in my mind that monitoring my progress with some notes has been not only therapeutic, it has clearly identified where I have noticed the biggest progress and that is the severity and reduction of skull pain and especially so while in a vehicle.

"My patience is wearing thin, as it has been for a long time. The only way I can stay positive is to reflect on where I have been, where I am at, and be forever hopeful that there is yet further progress to be made."

Regressive days back-to-back would strain and drain all of my resources. It did not matter how much I knew about self-management of pain; when it rules, it literally overrules everything in its way.

In early November we went to another theatre performance: "It is almost beyond comprehension to be able to see a performance, enjoy it, and not be fighting excruciating pain. Without a doubt things are progressing very favourably, albeit with the help of medication. However, the degree of pain is monumentally decreased."

It was obvious I was feeling better, but I was also thinking about what a serious setback the July 1991 accident had been. "As I am getting better, noticeably so, I cannot help but have serious feelings about how the July 1991 accident set me back. It has been a very traumatic experience. One that I could have done without. I am grateful for the fact that somehow I accepted my fate and did not let myself fall apart. It is hard to say that I will never recover those lost years as never is a strong word, however, *it is never*. Financially, it is a disaster. How does one measure compensation for the pain and suffering which I have endured, let alone the tremendous losses for my not working. And, at the stage I am in, a dilemma as to how soon I will be allowed to return to work."

On the odd occasion the thought occurred to me, "What if we had not moved to the country?" If we had not moved to the country, I would not have been where I was when the July 1991 accident occurred. I probably would have been back to work by this time. However, I quickly dispelled thoughts of "what if" as there was nothing I could do about the past. Fate was what brought us to the country and I accepted everything that went with it – what choice did I have?

On November 12, the day after Armistice Day, my diary reads: "Lest we Forget, yesterday was a day of remembrance for those who so valiantly fought for their country...For me, I cannot help but think of how much meaning these words, lest we forget, have for the living. Having gone through a very prolonged, traumatic health period, I cannot help but think of which friends rallied at the time of my distress. To be certain, it was both appreciated and overwhelming.

"However, as time goes by and one's illness is prolonged, the lest we forget syndrome sets in. You are in a different lifestyle and for the busy living, life goes on and yes, they do forget. If they do not forget, what they fail to do is keep in touch.

"It is ironic how much of a giver you can be, how much the public at large can be takers as long as you are there to give, and how you can fall by the wayside. My observations are not restricted to my experience only. I have had many occasions over the years to find people who are in distress to be very lonely."

During my years in active business life, I had often tried to put some joy into a person's life when he or she was down. I could easily have taken the attitude that I was too busy, but there was always such a fulfillment with the thanks I got. On one occasion an individual even requested that I visit him on his deathbed, wishing to see me once again to thank me for all that I had done. At that time, at that moment, I felt I had done so little.

There are so many people, ill, disabled, even healthy, who could use a visit. It could put a ray of light in their lives if we were to make the effort to spend time with them, and it could put a ray in our lives as well.

In late November the healing process continued. "Although I have the ability to look after myself, my body virtually controls me. The master role has changed and I desperately want to regain control. The pain is what keeps me like a horse in reins. You are a prisoner of your own body rather than the system, where a prisoner is monitored with some device. I am determined to overcome and in fact I believe I have - I must *HEAL*.

"I am still looking for a good day. A good day would be getting up with no pain and having such a day, all day. I am, however, grateful for the better days which I am experiencing.

"Certainly I knew what pain was, a bruise, a cut, a sting, you name it. However, within minutes, hours, or a few days the pain is gone. A sliver so small can cause so much pain, fester. Remove it and within a day or two healing has taken place. Fix the problem, attend to it, and you are well.

"What?? is so difficult with a facet joint? Do a facet block and you have relief. It wears off and I am back to square one.

"It is so slow. Why? What is the medication doing to me, besides giving me some relief? What is it doing to my gut? Surely there must be some quicker fix. Men can go to the moon but can't fix a facet joint."

I had learned that you can't push a body. It heals at its own speed, just as a river flows at its own speed and can't be pushed. It continued to be a difficult period with wide fluctuations of pain levels subdued by medication. There was no quick, permanent fix.

Fortunately I had varied interests that gave me the necessary distraction and willpower to carry on coping with adversity. I had positive thinking. And I had hope. In early December I watched a television program on health. A doctor ended the program by talking about hope in a patient. He stated that if a person gave up hope, they were dead. I had never associated hope with death, but as I reflected on the statement I had no doubt that I had never given up hope. There were many days, month to month, year to year, where things looked hopeless, but I never gave up hope that I would get better and I do believe the positive thoughts of hope helped keep me together. And now we lived about thirty minutes by car from a village called Hope.

In early December I wrote: "The last few months have been very strange. The variables, however, are that I am having more fair days rather than bad, difficult ones. A measuring rod which is so easily identified is my ability to hold my head backwards without excruciating pain. Yes, there is still pain radiating to the skull when I do so, however, it is at that moment. At this stage based on what is happening *it is time* and I must have the patience to wait, always in the hope that things are going in the right direction. I pray that things on the inside are an indication of healing and not just relief from medication."

During an early morning walk on a crisp and clear frosty morning, I heard and saw an interesting sight. A large flock of honking geese passed overhead. It was music to the ears, a sound of its own. About five minutes after the flock had passed, I heard a weak honk. I searched the sky and there was the straggler, making its way with great difficulty. I had on more than one occasion seen two or three together, separated from the rest, but never one by itself.

In December I experimented with various levels and variations of medication, all with no success. In my diary I asked, "Is this just another plateau or is this *the* plateau?" Various activities continued to put me in a regressive state, but the recovery period was not as prolonged. I found with my bowling that "the intensity of the pain now develops towards the end of the first game. This is a marked change from the beginning of the season when I was in deep trouble after having thrown just a few balls." It was encouraging and yet I was still discouraged with every setback. If I had no control over the pain, I had the control of continually fighting back.

In the third week of December I had further cortisone injections in the back of the skull area for the trapezius muscle. That area continued to be tender and inflamed.

Once more I asked Dr. Bull what he thought about my getting back to work. He said he felt my condition would not improve too much in the future, that I was about as good as I would get, and that it was a matter of how well I could cope if I returned to work.

All along, this was where my heart had been; I wanted to get back to work. Over the years I had developed other interests to keep me occupied till the day I would get back to work. However, I was not elated by the doctor's comments. I knew I was making slow but positive progress and he was being realistic about my prospects. If I went back to work, I'd still need to cope with pain.

On December 25 my diary reads: "As I reflect on where I was a year ago, I have come a long way. Even though I have strength, act strong, have faith, trust, belief, hope, love, and a deep conviction that I will overcome, the debilitating health problem has me in its clutches.

"I hope and pray that the wide fluctuations in pain levels on almost a daily basis are positive healing, if this is what healing is all about. For certain, I do have some relief as compared to intensive pain previously, twenty-four hours a day.

"It is a great day. We have family with us. A daughter, three sons, a daughter- and son-in-law, and five grandchildren. Eleven in all, the largest Christmas family gathering in many years."

This was the sixth Christmas since my surgery in December 1988. Little did I know at that time what was in store for me.

On New Year's Eve we entertained some good friends, Chris and Bob. On a number of occasions Bob had talked about how you go through life and end up with a handful of what may be referred to as true friendships. Our visit made me reflect on the many people and friendships we have over a lifetime. During the ten years of my health problems it often seemed that someone I had not heard from for some time would give me a call or drop in. We crave friendships whether we are healthy or not. I cannot recall being lonesome during my period of disability. In fact, in troubled times I was not good company in any event and best left alone. When you are not well it can be a full-time job to look after yourself. There are times when you welcome visitors and then there are times when you would prefer others not see how you are suffering. Everyone understands this.

However, what I wish to stress is that if you are not well and are craving contact, call a friend and invite him or her for a visit. If you are unable to pick up the phone to invite someone over yourself, get someone to do it for you. When you are not well, all too often your friends do not know how to deal with you. Give them a call and let them know you are ready for visitors. Do it now.

My diary shows we had visitors in our home an average of two times a week. When our grandchildren visited I would take them hiking, bowling, or to the golf driving range – activities that were enjoyable but were also, for me, a form of therapy. Going for a drive was always a measure of how I was or was not progressing. Over the years I also did not lack for visits with doctors and medical laboratories. In 1993 I visited with my personal physician and other specialists on eighteen occasions and had ten lab reports.

I maintained my interest in elephant garlic and from 300 cloves planted, harvested 1050 cloves. It was a small piece of ground for me to look after, but it was something to keep me busy and it gave me a great feeling of accomplishment when the garlic was harvested. I also planted my first crop of gourds. I had always marvelled at the gourds

206

when they showed up in stores around Thanksgiving time and would bring a few home for Sasha, so this year I thought I would grow my own. There were not many seeds in each package, so I thought I had better get several packets in case some of them did not grow. Much to my surprise there were plants from all the hills, and I did not thin any of them out. As the vines grew, then blossomed, I knew I was going to have more than a few gourds, and it was wonderful to go to the gourd patch and look at the various shapes and colours developing. At harvest time, Sasha not only had more gourds than ever before, but every visitor to our home took some. I could not believe it: 250 gourds from a few packages of seeds.

The year was not without its difficult periods. There were many changes in my condition, and change brought a lot of concern about what was really happening to me. Throughout these periods of change and new stresses I did my best to remain as active as possible within my limitations – or perhaps it's better to say I was as active as possible to the limits of my capabilities. But when I reviewed the year's activities, I wondered how I had time for anything other than not being well.

There was no question that my health problem had a grip on me and that, had I allowed it to happen, it would have consumed all of my time as well. Fortunately I have always looked at time as a precious commodity and I could not see myself wasting all of my time due to my health. I must, however, qualify this statement. There were periods when all of my time was consumed by my health and when I was working overtime just to keep up. Throughout the year I practised pain-management techniques on a daily basis. What was showing through the cracks was that I was starting to have positive results from some of them or that healing was taking its course – probably both.

"I hope and pray that these positive signs continue. It is as if it were a new beginning to experience so much relief. I believe more than ever that I have reached another plateau and I will continue all my disciplines reaching for the next one."

Chapter 18

TEN YEARS

The original car accident that started my health ordeal took place in November 1984, so I was now approaching the tenth anniversary of the accident. Ten years is a long time to be suffering from a rear-ender that had not seemed to be too serious. What was serious was the impact, which actually bent the frame on the car. If you bend metal, what effect can you expect it to have on your body?

When I consider how long I dealt with this health problem, I marvel at how I was able to continue the faith. On January 29, 1994, my diary starts out; "Clear skies, a beautiful morning, days are noticeably longer. Yesterday I did some pruning of blackberry bushes, a branch at a time, a couple of hours and the speed is slow, however, like the hare and the tortoise there is a message. Do what you can, there is a lot of gratification in doing something, no matter how little, but it is daily and preserves my sanity. Hopefully this positive trend continues, and I will be exploring my options of getting back to work."

Perhaps the word faith is important as when all else has failed, we still have time if we only believe that things are slowly changing. The body may be responding to treatment and relaxation, though it is not noticeable. It is not noticeable until one day, in a strange and subtle way, you find there is a small change in your condition – and without a doubt faith played a part. The change may be so small that it takes several days, weeks, months, even years before it becomes noticeable in your daily routine. One day it would seem I was on my way out of pain and then just as fast I would be back to square one. On good days I would write, "Is this really true? Is this really happening to me? Can I really be feeling quite good in the morning and down and out by evening?" When the change was in my favour I swallowed it up. Why shouldn't I? After ten years of suffering, a little relief was a lot. But then I would regress and wonder if my body was playing dirty tricks on me. Eventually I learned they were not dirty tricks; the name of the game was healing, slow and steady.

At times there was an element of doubt as I wondered if I was making the right decision in a given situation. As I slowly got better I became more confident about my self-management. I had more faith in my ability to look after myself than I'd had in earlier times when I was literally crying for help twenty-four hours a day. There were many times I feared that something new was creeping in, but now that I knew what pain was about I would handle it on my own instead of making a trip to the emergency room. After the bowling sessions there were many times when I could have gone straight to the doctor's office or to emergency, but this is where I learned to self-manage and hope that there was not something new happening.

I can recall one of my specialists remarking, "There is no quick fix." I still wonder why he did not elaborate on what kind of fix there might be. It would have been most reassuring if he had said, "It may take a long time," or if he had even identified the time period and given me some assurance that there was a possibility I would improve considerably. If only he had said, "A body, and especially the head area, is not built for impacts such as you have had. There can be a lot of damage, but as long as you work at it and have a lot of patience, with time things may settle down." Maybe in his own words he said this, but if he did, I did not hear them. I was left to manage myself in a condition that seemed hopeless at the time, struggling to survive on a daily basis. Of course this is what happens to all of us when we are unwell. The medical profession helps as much as it can, but the rest lies squarely on our own shoulders.

I do not know how I rose to the occasion and continued to fight a battle of pain. Everyone at one time or another has experienced pain, but you do not know what pain is until you have lived with it for twenty-four hours a day for years. I was relying on medical specialists to help me get well, but when they could not fix me up they directed me to other specialists who would teach me how to better manage the pain.

For me, the term "pain management" has a negative tone. I did not want to learn how to better manage the pain. I was already managing it. What I wanted was to get rid of the pain and get on with life. (I can understand that some people might need help learning how to manage pain. I am all for providing help and learning how to cope with pain. But I am also for getting rid of the pain.)

I sincerely believe I am coming from the deepest depths of pain. I would never question another person or doubt their claim that they had suffered or were suffering from pain. It is one of the most debilitating forces around and it took a tremendous amount of effort to weather the storm. Unlike a usual storm that settles after a day or two, this one raged day in and day out for years on end and held me in a grip so strong that I had no one to turn to. It took a lot of self-talk to convince me that I could hold myself together until someone was able to help me, although it often seemed that, medically, I was in the dark ages.

It was difficult to face the reality of a health problem from year to year, but it was also difficult to understand why it dragged on. I could not comprehend why, with advanced medical technology, I had to be subjected to such prolonged suffering. I thought there must be many former patients in whose footsteps I was following for treatment. Surely doctors had identified patterns that indicated how various individuals were affected and how they healed. I wondered why the specialist did not share more thoughts and information with me. I was hungry to know the answers. I wanted to be told where I was at and what were my chances of getting better.

The unknown was the most difficult aspect to deal with and I was overwhelmed by unknowns. My philosophy, as I've mentioned before, was if you have a problem you must find it, fix it, and get on with life. Unfortunately, in the medical field it is not as simple as a diagnosis and a quick fix. There are too many possible causes or contributing factors, and the patient must continue to endure while the medical profession sorts them out – if it can be sorted out. If I had been told about potential problems and if my specialists had outlined how we were going to approach them, one by one, I would at least have received some peace of mind. Instead, medical people wrote letters to other medical people about my case, but I was not given the opportunity to read them (and I would not have understood the medical terminology at that time in any event). Perhaps I was not aggressive enough about asking for the answers, but when you are down and out, how aggressive can you be? When you are "filled with drugs which left me a walking zombie," as I wrote in my diary, how can you be aggressive and ask questions?

Perhaps time was the problem. I had a lot of time and it was survival time, but perhaps the medical people were too caught up with heavy patient loads. Maybe there should be an understudy working alongside these busy people, someone who can carry the slack between patient and specialist.

On the other hand, I remember one specialist who could not help me who said, "Go home and continue to do whatever it is you are doing. Do not get on a treadmill of seeing specialists. They cannot help you." It was strong advice and by the time I was referred to this specialist, that was precisely what I was doing. I'd put in place a complete-as-possible self-management program on my own.

Even though I told myself that I would get better, I do not believe this reassurance was strongly transmitted to me by those who were caring for me. I recognize that it might not be the best idea to build false hopes when dealing with the unknown. I do recall how my orthopaedic surgeon once stated, "If it's the last thing I do, I am going to fix you up." When he made the statement, little did we know how significant his vow was, as he himself was having medical problems and shortly after my second surgery he had to leave his practice due to a disability. I will be forever grateful to that man. I also must say that in spite of my reservations, I was impressed with the majority of help I received. I had great respect for the various procedures attempted and the practitioners I dealt with and I could not have done without them. The one thing I could have done without was the strange neurological examination that left me with welts on my back from the fist pounding.

One of the specialists I saw many years before had compared the healing process to a ball of wool. He told me, "You have a difficult problem to deal with. In addition to the serious neck problem there is the multitude of neck muscles, nerves, and nerve endings which have been disrupted." He wanted me to think of my neck area as a ball of wool that had been unwound. "After unravelling it, I would like you to think of putting it back together exactly the way it was."

My response was that it would be impossible, but he replied that, with time and all going well, my body might heal on its own. "I wish

I could give you more words of encouragement," he concluded, "but this is the best I can do."

Now, in 1994, it felt like the ball of wool was coming back together. "It is looking good. I am tolerating pain, BUT IT IS ON MY OWN. I hope and pray that it keeps up. There are definitely signs of another plateau. Incredible as it may seem, I was in a very deep gully, slowly but surely recovering, always looking for the top, reaching for new plateaus, sliding back when you least expect it, forever believing I will reach the summit and I believe I am near."

The significance of tolerating pain "ON MY OWN" was that I had been able to break the cycle of taking medication on a regular basis. I still had days when it was uncomfortable, as if the pain were going to come on strong. "It is disheartening, to say the least, however, unlike in the past, I think what I will do is rather than put up with the lingering pain, take some medication on the occasion of pain and on increasing pain. It is a killer and even though I want to do without medication, I cannot let pride stand in my way." I also knew that a day or two of medication would give me immediate relief and carry me for a while. My days were so much better. I had learned to tolerate and manage a lot of pain, but I was still searching for that pain-free day, not knowing whether I would ever have one in the future. And at this point, if I stayed at status quo, I knew I could manage. I recognized that I had come a long way. "This is of course markedly different from before when there was virtually no noticeable relief. In my layperson's opinion, I had built very high tolerance levels for pain and now some of my self-management techniques are actually showing results as long as I continue to have a lot of patience. Self-management of pain takes time, commitment, and a never fading hope that good will come out of it."

Further positive reinforcement came from people like Dr. Sookochoff, my urologist. I had an annual check-up with him in February and he observed how much better I looked. He had been seeing me for a number of years, saw me at my worst, and now he recognized a big change since the previous year's visit. It was one thing when people had contact with me on a regular basis; it was another when they saw me once a year and noticed the change in my condition. That was encouraging. (I can also recall how gentle, courteous, and understanding these same people were when they saw me in troubled times. I was embarrassed deep inside when I showed signs of not being well. I tried not to show it or talk about it, but I also could not apologize for the way people saw me. I always knew when I was down and out, and if a visitor mentioned he or she thought I was a little offbeat, I was quite willing to admit it was because I was not having one of my better days. Although I did not know what it was to have a better day, I found that people were most understanding when I told them and was open about it.)

The other interesting aspect was that people who saw me on a periodic basis were commenting on how much weight I had lost. Many thought my weight loss was due to the prolonged illness. "It sure took a lot out of you, didn't it?" they would say. I always assured them that the weight loss was by design, and I felt deep satisfaction whenever someone commented on it. This showed my Commitment to Health program was successful and it vindicated my dedication to good diet and aerobic walking.

There was always progress to report. On January 12, 1994, for example: "Drove myself to bowling yesterday. The bowling experience continues to be precisely that, an experience pain wise which I could do without. On the positive side, there is a decrease in pain while bowling until about the eighth frame in the first game. After that it is living torture. In spite of this, yesterday, I bowled my best game of the year, a two-hundred and eighty-four, the first and last games were a disaster."

On January 30 we drove to Vancouver where we met friends for lunch and then attended a live theatre matinee performance. "It was a wonderful get together. Everyone enjoyed the outing. Sasha loved it. For me it was a fair day, and especially so when you consider the drive, meeting for lunch, the play, and then for a coffee after the show. As I reflected on the day, what was most significant was the reduction in the level of pain endured during the performance. A similar outing in the past was nothing short of an endurance exercise, managing the compounded pain. Yesterday, although not without additional pain during the performance, it was not as intense as in the past, the pain was with me the rest of the day, however the intensity of the compounded pain was measurably reduced. To say the least, I am pleased with the progress."

On February 11: "As I write these notes, I do have some neck pain, gripping, radiating to the skull. However, there is, I hope, some very positive good news. Yesterday I drove myself to visit mother, had lunch with one of my sons in Vancouver, and before leaving for home, although not without some compounded neck pain, I was not much worse off than before I had left.

"Moreover, by the time I got home around five p.m., I was not in compounded pain such that I could not tolerate on my own. I did not take any additional medication for relief and by bedtime things had settled to status quo levels. What a revelation to have things settle down the same day.

"I could scream for joy to think that I was in this type of recovery before the July 1991 accident. It was, to say the least, a traumatic setback."

In mid-April I wrote, "The bowling session was precisely that, a session. Of particular noticeable interest was that the compounded pain did not come on until the third game, at which time the skull pain was quite strong." I remember how I felt on that day – in pain but elated. The difference between being in severe compounded pain early in the first game, which is how things were when I started bowling, and what I had just experienced seemed like another miracle in my progress to better health and reduced pain.

On April 18: "Yesterday we had a group of former school friends out for brunch. For me, what was very positive was that I was able to enjoy the visit without excruciating pain. Yes, I am and was tolerating some pain. However, by the end of the day I was not in compounded pain. Without question I am standing up much better to the rigours of a day."

This was another milestone, a significant one. Instead of sitting off to the side minding my own pain, I was able to mingle. I would not have imagined before 1984 that I could be so disabled that I would cut a visit short or not even attend a social function because of my pain. Now it was a revelation, and in some ways a trauma, to be in a social environment, whether one on one or in a group, and not suffer the consequences of a severe setback at the end of the day. Suddenly I was overcome with thoughts of, "What is going on? I am not fighting pain." Fighting and managing pain had become a full-time job, and anytime you are in a full-time job you must give it your best in order to succeed. It rested on my shoulders to make the most of each and every situation. I had given it my best and now the job was disappearing. I did not have to spend hours on end self-managing high pain levels.

For me, writing about a positive event continued to be a form of therapeutic healing. Writing about the negatives was also a positive reinforcement. It was good to put them in writing and get them out of my mind for the moment. Instead of getting drowned in my troubles, as it would have been easy to do, I never let my mind dwell on the negative. For every negative I would let my creative mind dwell on positive things to do within my limitations, things that would help overrule the negatives.

I did everything I could to avoid negative self-talk throughout the day. I may have let up at times for a day or two when I was seriously stricken, but I never gave up hope. When you are on your own, becoming skilled at pain management, it is not easy to maintain high hopes of recovery. But these high hopes must have top priority in your mind and your self-talk. You have to believe beyond a doubt that you are getting well and will be better. It may seem like you are feeding yourself garbage, but I would much sooner feed myself positive garbage than negative. And when you do, make certain you write it down.

With this reduction in pain came the need to adjust my activities commensurate with my increased abilities. It was like skating on thin ice. If you have never skated on thin ice on a pond in winter, you won't be familiar with the sound of crackling and the sudden sight of long crack marks across the ice surface. It is scary and I was finding that cracks might not show up until a day or two after an activity. The cracks often occurred after self-induced punishment, like my bowling sessions.

Through my difficult periods of rehabilitation I had held the philosophy "No pain, no gain." This philosophy was not shared by all. Physiotherapists had strong words of caution against continuing an exercise when it caused noticeable pain. They would stress that as soon as it started to hurt I should stop and leave it for another day, then build on it from day to day as my body allowed during the healing process.

Over the years I heard both sides and I came to believe that if I was able to carry out an exercise, I should do it – our bodies were made for it. I had to have patience, but I always liked the saying of my orthopaedic surgeon: "Use it or lose it." I saw how this applied to my circumstances after my first surgery. Instead of using my neck and building up the muscles, I was continually restricting them with a cervical collar. I had to use the collar after surgery to stabilize the fusion, but the prolonged use of the collar caused the neck muscles to atrophy and I lost the strength of my neck.

One activity I did not give up was my aerobic walking. On June 23, 1994, I wrote: "As I further reflect, perhaps the one greatest factor which has helped me to get where I am is the 'Commitment to Health,' which I made in 1984. Walking, I walked the hills and sea wall in our prior neighbourhood and now I walk the hill of our country road daily.

"My progress is most gratifying. The discipline of walking, rain or shine, is precisely that, a discipline. Now it is such that it is a part of my daily life, a routine which my body actually craves and I believe the healthiest for you. I often wonder, as a percentage of the population, how many are able to dedicate themselves to such a firm regimen over a prolonged period of time.

"I will be forever grateful that I took the time to make it a daily discipline and I can guarantee that anyone who may wish to do the same can, no matter how busy they may think and/or believe they are. One of these days I shall track Dr. [Ken] Cooper down, give him a call, and express my appreciation of what he did for me."

Better eating habits and daily walking were both part of my full-time pain-fighting job. During the ten years we always resided about a third of the way up a mountainside. When we lived in the city, my daily walks took me over hilly terrain. Our move to the country meant considerable uphill and downhill walking every day. My pace may not have been up to speed-walking standards, but at least I was walking and not being pushed in a wheelchair.

Even though I would add to the pain with every step, walking was a way to pass the time. Perhaps the desire to get up and go for walks so frequently was a sign of boredom. If it was, I did not recognize it as such. What I did recognize and hope was that I was doing something right for my body – a continuation of my Commitment to Health program.

There is only an "i" and "n" separating activity and inactivity, but what a tremendous difference in meaning and in lifestyle. To be active requires a commitment whether you are healthy or not – for the individual who is not healthy it is that much more of a commitment. If you are unwell, "activity" may not be the right word. I found it too straightforward, harsh, demanding. It left me feeling I had to do something, but when I was at my lowest points I did not want to be burdened with activity. This is where mind over matter played a big role. The size of the activity was unimportant. What mattered was the self-disciplined desire to do something constructive each and every day, no matter how menial.

Listing on paper the activities I wanted to do was a better approach. This was a form of brain activity and I came up with many worthwhile endeavours that became important to me. When I put the idea into writing, I created activity in a subtle way – it was something I wanted to do, not something I felt I had to do. The important thing was to be as active as I could be; it was too easy to be inactive. I stretched myself as much as I could without hurting myself and discovered that the ability to carry on in the most difficult circumstances is vital and valuable (and is usually not tapped at all by healthy individuals).

Anyone faced with a debilitating health setback should get to know and understand the limitations set by the health condition. Do not allow yourself to be fenced in, boxed in. Realize that such situations have a way of getting control of your life and controlling you. Illness can have an overwhelming strength and will get you in its clutches so strongly that you could face a major problem trying to get untangled.

Every day everyone is being tested in one form or another. These tests are the means by which we learn to get by in the world. The test of managing pain – prolonged, unrelenting pain, often referred to as chronic pain – is a learning experience. I believe it is one of the most difficult situations an individual may ever have to live with. You cannot beat it, but if you accept it for what it is you can learn to deal with it and manage it so that it does not have you totally in its clutches.

As I wrote in February 1994: "It is a strange plateau I am in, if you could call it that. However, on reflection, this trade-off is certainly welcome over that of twenty-four hours a day excruciating pain. It has and continues to take a lot of something, determination, courage, sticktoitiveness – you name it, I need it...I have been and continue to be tested to the nth degree, to limits which I never knew I had within me, limits of a different kind."

Perhaps another way of putting it is you do not need mind over matter but matter over mind. When you are suffering from chronic pain, pain that leaves you crying for help, mind over matter will not help. Relaxation techniques may help you achieve a sense of calm (though I used to ask myself how much more relaxation I needed, as that was all I was doing for days, months, and years) but will not eliminate the pain. I lived, breathed, and managed myself at the speed dictated by my body. Any other speed was not compatible with the pain. When I ventured outside my boundaries and my body was not ready for it, my body put me in my place. It was a strange phenomenon to adjust to, particularly for a former workaholic, but I believe it would be tough for anyone under similar circumstances.

Instead, I was fortunate because I was eventually able to get back to driving, going out on my own to get a haircut, to buy some groceries at the store, or to buy fresh fruit and vegetables at the farmers' market – to distract myself with things in the real world outside my mind. It didn't make the pain go away, but gave me something to think about besides the pain. I led an adjusted lifestyle within my limitations, but I did live and I am most grateful I did so.

It was hard for me to accept that everything I did must be for myself. I had to maintain a selfish point of view. If ever there was a time I felt carved out from the rest of the world, it was in my darkest moments. Yet I simply created my own world, which I lived and revolved in. I have no doubt that my personal applications and dedication to helping myself get better with outside projects allowed me to get through each and every day.

It truly was a full-time job, but how different from my former job. As time went on I would think about the great preparation I used to go through when there was a holiday weekend with three days off work. With my disability, Sasha and I were often taken by surprise when we came upon a long holiday weekend. We were engrossed by my problem and although we rated a weekend off, I did not qualify. I was left with no choice but to live in my world as best I could. Just for a moment, think of someone telling you that for the next ten years you will not be entitled to statutory holiday pay or to your two-week vacation. We do not live that way, but if you are a victim of crunching metal and if your body does not respond to a healing process, that is the situation you will be in. You lose your career, your job and its benefits. Life-saving self-management techniques become your new career, though you get no wages or benefits from this full-time job. Self-management becomes crisis management and when you are dealing with crisis management under ordinary living circumstances, you are carrying a heavy load.

I could dwell on how it destroyed my career, but I am so grateful and fortunate to be able to say it did not totally destroy me. It could have destroyed me if it had all happened at once, but it did not. I knew there was something wrong as I was not myself from the day of the original accident, but the deterioration was slow. It took years to reach the lowest point and in those years there were adjustment periods when I learned to live with a progressively worsening health condition. This slow deterioration allowed me to somehow adjust to and manage the condition.

There is no question I went through difficult times, not least when I left behind a business enterprise built on giving it everything you have got. However, I knew that as long as I had my faculties about me I could start a new venture on recovery. I might have been more worried if I had been told, "You are finished, you will never return to work," but this is not what I was told.

If I had been told, "It will be ten years or more before you are recovered. Consider yourself retired," I would have been devastated – more devastated than I was already. However, again, I was not told that. At first there was a chance to get back to work in six months and then, as time and fate would have it, the disability dragged on, our lifestyle changed, my interest in life was sustained, and when the reality that I would be off work for some time set in, fate of another kind came along and we made a move to a new residence. We had not planned to move from where we were, but over the years I have come to respect the word "never." It is such a definite, certain word, or so it seems to me. I know that I am cautious about using the word "never" because never in my wildest thoughts or dreams would I ever have believed what happened to me.

All it took was a split second to destroy a concrete set of plans to a known destination and to start a new journey to a world of the unknown for ten years. I knew where I was going. I knew how fast I was growing in my business. I knew, I knew, I knew!

As it turned out, it mattered not how much I knew. What mattered was what I did not know. Enter the world of the unknown, the world of the serious medical problem. It is difficult enough to deal with medical problems. In my case, the problem was compounded because there were no definitive answers.

I had no way of knowing what fate had in store for me. It is a blessing that we live in a world of the unknown.

I was fifty-three years of age at the time of my accident in 1984. As I write this chapter in 1995 I have just turned sixty-four years of age. If I were healthy I would be thinking of retirement one year away, as it was mandatory at age sixty-five under my contract.

Instead, I had my career carved out from under me. But over the ten-year period I carved out a rehabilitation career of which I am proud, not so much for what I accomplished as for the mere fact that I was able to accomplish it. I have done many things during these ten years that in all likelihood I would not have done under normal circumstances.

Over the years I have met many people who have had both health and other types of problems and all too often they ask, "Why did this have to happen to me?"

It is a difficult question to answer. I believe there is no answer other than, "That's life" or "That's fate." We cannot go around feeling sorry for ourselves. We must pull things together and, if necessary, slowly create a new lifestyle as I did. If we do not get that pen and paper and start writing out our concerns, I can, based on my experience and contact with others over the years, almost guarantee that self-pity is going to cause setback and slower recovery. The key is to get on with life and do it now as best you can.

It was fate that I suffered the two car accidents, but it was also fate that I opened the classified section of our daily paper and read an ad about a piece of property that was to change our lives. Fate forced me to give up many of the things I enjoyed doing – my job, coaching young people in sports, community work, and personal sports activities like swimming – but fate also brought me, many years earlier, to meet my wife Sasha at a Halloween dance, a wonderful fate. The past decade was difficult for both of us, but was also memorable, filled with change.

If you can allow the word faith to come into your life along with fate, it could well be that the faith will blend in with whatever fate you face. Faith in self and faith in others will pull you through.

On July 14 I heard of the death of a woman we knew. Apparently she had a difficult time after her husband died three months earlier. She became depressed and lost the will to live. I thought of the tremendous strength I often had to call on and how I was literally on my deathbed many times. I believe I came out of it because I had the will, the power, and the willpower to fight adversity at a level I had never experienced in my lifetime. It would have been so easy to give up, but I had much to live for: my wife, my children, my grandchildren, nature, which all too often we take for granted, the smell of the flowers, the singing of the birds, and the eagles soaring overhead.

I learned I had to get my priorities in order, get a handle on the problem, figure out what I could do about it, figure out what others could do about it, and most important, get all of my concerns in writing and start those projects and activities that were going to help keep me occupied.

Before my accident I had never had the opportunity to literally waste time. After my accident I had to accept that if I could putter daily, the time frame did not matter. What mattered was the feeling of accomplishment, of doing something. The problem was I had a whole day to get rid of but I was only good for some puttering time, so it took a high degree of discipline to be satisfied with doing so little. Particularly with gardening, there were many times when I would be weeding, down on my hands and knees, one weed at a time, feeling so sick that I would ask myself why I was doing it. Did I not have something better to do?

The answers came quickly. I was doing it because, within my limitations, it was something I could do as long as I persevered.

Nothing more and nothing less. It was a project to help me get through my day on a periodic weeding basis. It was not easy, but then nothing is. Once I started something, I had to bring the project to completion. In some ways my health was the same.

Menial activity became a way of charting my progress. On July 21, 1994, I wrote: "Yesterday I weeded and hoed the garden and if I were to go back to a year ago, I was pulling weeds on my hands and knees and in absolute pain. Now I can hoe bending over and not endure a lot of compounded pain.

"I am now managing on two medications, except for the odd difficult day and these are becoming both infrequent and most positive in that a day or two of anti-inflammatory medication settles things down."

I learned to be grateful for doing a little, and when those little accomplishments were spread out over time they turned out to be a lot. You need self-management and self-discipline. You need to know when to start and, more importantly, when to stop.

I had the same quantity of time as everyone else, but that twenty-four hours took on a different meaning. In a normal day the average working person performs a variety of tasks. The same held true for me. In my world I got up just like everyone else, had my meals for the day, made the best of every day, and went on to the next day. However, my world differed from the norm because it was filled with pain from sun up to sun down as well as through the night, day in and day out, stretching into months and years. Pain can make that quantity of sixty minutes drag on for what seems like hours. When you are lying on your back for days, it is incredible how slowly time will pass. My environment was, for the most part, the confines of my home and property. I was free to go anywhere I wanted at any time with no restrictions other than the ones my body imposed on me. These were enough to make me stay indoors and become a prisoner not only of my body but also of our home. For this reason I did my best to come up with things I could do to help get rid of the quantity of time I had on my hands. Even getting out for a walk gave me some quality time. Adding quality to the minutes and hours was most important. We must be aware that both quality and quantity of time are at our disposal and must make the most of them.

When I stayed indoors it was not easy to redirect my thought processes away from the heavy burden of pain. I was still burdened when I went outdoors for my walk, but there was a diversion, a mind-clearing exercise that set my thoughts flowing on a new track. I do know that when I was walking, I was careful to have a balance between the positive and negative influences that were going on in my life. For a long time the negative influence predominated, and it was during this time that I found walking to be most helpful to me. The negative of pain did not disappear (in fact, most of the time I would end up having compounded pain as with every step there was additional pain radiating to the skull), but there was a distraction from it. Most obviously, there were always things to observe in the world around me as I walked. This was a benefit of walking that goes beyond the physical benefit.

Slowly but surely the unknown status of my health started to turn to the known. I was getting better. This was the ultimate goal: to start getting better and to continue doing everything I could to help myself along the way. It was encouraging and satisfying to record the improvements. I was satisfied because I had not given up and also because it seemed that every time I made some notes I could compare the past and the present and see the changes that were so significant in the tenth year. On July 5 I wrote: "Most interesting is that the progress has been so noticeable this year as compared to the past where it was at a snail's pace and I could not help but wonder as to whether or not I would reach higher plateaus of health." And on July 6: "If I were to make as much progress in the next three to six months as I have year to date, I will be enjoying a much higher standard of health."

Through most of the decade of my health problem I thought in terms of one-year periods. As I started to get noticeably better in 1994, time frames became shorter and I found I could record progress on a day-to-day basis. If I slipped backwards after reaching another plateau, the recovery was noticeably quicker. Things would settle the same day or overnight. I no longer had to go through days of coping until the pain had settled down.

Another miracle, admittedly slow in coming, was my ever-improving ability to tolerate pain as a driver or a passenger in a vehicle. I would have a twinge of pain radiating to the skull, but this was a marked improvement over my previous condition when there was excruciating compounded pain radiating to the skull.

My life had been made up of endless visits to doctors, but now I saw only my personal physician on a monthly basis for a check-up. It was a welcome relief not to be continually going to medical appointments. Although appointments are generally quite brief, they do carve up the days, especially when travel is involved. It took me the better part of a day to travel to Vancouver for appointments. As I got better, so much time was freed up for me – time I had to fill with other activities.

I knew I was not out of the woods as I had been told I would always be left with some level of disability. Bone spurs, scar tissue, and inflammation would cause discomfort I would have to live with. I could never expect to be 100 percent. The guessing game in the tenth year was to estimate where I would plateau. I wanted to find out what I was up against for the rest of my life. As I charted my progress, it was most encouraging. I was not without some problems, but it appeared the real heavy ones were behind me.

Now that one long-term problem was dissipating, however, another moved forward to take my attention. The pain in my right hip had been getting progressively worse. X-rays taken early in 1994 showed some bone spurs, but other than that everything seemed to be alright. I found it difficult to believe but accepted the reading. In November more X-rays were taken. Dr. Bull told me these X-rays showed that the joint space in the hip had narrowed since the beginning of the year. The diagnosis was osteoarthritis. The hip could either stabilize or become so badly worn that I would require a hip replacement. This hit me like a ton of bricks. I had been feeling so much better and here was a new condition to worry about.

I went to see a rheumatologist who said there was no question in her mind that I would require a hip replacement and that I should be seeing an orthopaedic surgeon. I asked how there could be such a change in ten months, but the rheumatologist said she had seen this type of condition develop quickly on previous occasions. It was not a good day but it was reassuring to know what the problem was. I was prescribed a cane and sent on my way.

Changes in the tenth year were slow and subtle, but also sure and certain. I could recognize that they were happening and I recorded many positive signs in my diary. There were difficult days, but they were far outnumbered by better days. I also enjoyed longer days. So much happened, yet it was not an overnight magic. I did not get to the point where I could say "I have recovered," but I could say, "What a difference ten years makes." It was as if I were coming out of a bad dream, but I was waking up to the fact that I was ten years older. That was scary. Ten years is a long time and in my case it was a career carve-out that I had no choice but to live with. No matter what happens, we never do have a choice but to live with it.

Through the year I did not deviate from any of my self-disciplined health management techniques. Self-management played such a big part in my recovery. At the end of the day – and for that matter at the beginning of each and every day – I was on my own. Everyone was sympathetic to my problem, but because I needed time to heal I was left to manage my pain and my daily life as best I could. Whatever I did was entirely up to me.

I had my self-management relaxation techniques; I read; I wrote; I kept a journal; I took photographs; I collected plates, native art, Mexican ironwood carvings, and antiques; I built model airplanes; I restored antique vehicles and a log building on our new property; I developed our fruit orchard and a Christmas tree plantation; I gardened. For the most part I had not planned to do these projects before my accident. They were put in place because I was a victim of circumstances far beyond my control, with only the self-knowledge and belief that with time I would get better.

I must give credit to those medical people who did not give up on me, although I must admit I was probably a difficult patient to look after. Not difficult to deal with as a person, but difficult because of the nature of the problem. I became much more a patient with patience as time went on. Patience is not easy to maintain, particularly when you see no progress in your health situation over a long period of time. But now I was seeing progress.

Last but not least I credit my Commitment to Health program. When I was assured that the problem in my spine would not interfere with my walking, I was relieved. This is not to say it was easy to continue walking, but with every step I felt a keen sense of accomplishment. I told myself that no matter what was going on, at least I could walk and I must be grateful for this.

I cannot ever expect to return to full health. However, I believe I am about as good as I will get and if I should get even better I will take all I can get. It was a long haul, but it was worth all the pain and suffering for the trade-off of being better. As well, I had the opportunity to grow from within in a manner I would never have thought possible. The reward of self-growth came from self-determination and self-discipline. It took ten years out of my life, but there is no doubt something went back in. There were many times when it would have been so easy to quit fighting, but what was the alternative? Had I allowed myself to drown in all of the negative health problems there could and probably would have been a different outcome.

It is hard to fathom a ten-year block of one's life. It is even hard for me to understand what I have gone through, but it is not a mystery. The facts are cold and revealing and I am certain that many have suffered or are suffering from similar trauma. I hope and pray that those who are presently suffering and those caregivers who are looking after them will find some sources of both comfort and inspiration from my account.

Although others may see you suffering from something beyond your power, believe in yourself and what your body is telling you. Draw on all of your human resources – there are many to draw on and you may need to tap into each and every one. Do not underestimate yourself, believe in who you are and what you stand for, love yourself as you have never loved before, believe in others and trust that they will help you, but do allow your creative mind to ask questions of those helping you if you are in doubt (with the understanding that maybe they have done or are doing everything they can for you), and always remember that you need time, maybe a lot of it.

Chapter 19

IS THERE A SUMMIT?

I know that many have preceded me in overcoming serious health problems resulting from motor vehicle accidents. There are many people who are presently suffering and many who have become quadri- or paraplegic from accidents. There are untold numbers of people who have suffered strokes, heart attacks, stress, and other disabling illnesses and conditions. The list is endless, and each person has a story to tell.

I hope that my story will be of use to people who have problems of various kinds, not just those who are recovering from a motor vehicle accident or a spinal problem. I believe that the chapter on my Commitment to Health will be of help to many on its own. When I started my Commitment I was so excited about my progress that I decided I would write a book on how you can take charge and, through the aerobics of walking and close monitoring of eating habits, get yourself back in shape. The book would be written under one condition: that I was successful with my Commitment to Health program.

As it turned out, my Commitment to Health program was in place and proving successful when I had my motor vehicle accident, which caused my overall health to regress. As time went on from months to years, I decided that my Commitment to Health was playing such a significant role in my overall health that I would change the original plan for the book, expanding it to cover how to deal with a long-term, debilitating condition.

It is now two years since I wrote the previous chapter. At that time I wrote that I believed I had reached the summit. There is now no question in my mind that I had reached a summit as far as my neck problems were concerned. Today my neck is literally problem free. It is as if nothing had ever happened to it – hard to believe when I consider the length of time I was not well.

The past two years have not been without further health problems, however. This has caused me to give a new definition to my idea of reaching the summit. During my extensive rehabilitation period I thought of my health as a mountain and my recovery as a climb. When I think of how many plateaus there were in getting better, I realize what a difficult ascent it was. There were also a lot of avalanches that would bury me or crevasses I would slip into for days, months, and years.

With every sign of relief I felt I was at another plateau, but I never reached a plateau and stayed there without slipping back. On many occasions, when I thought I was at a new plateau it turned out to be an illusion. The body gave me a taste of what was to come, but that was all it was. When it was ready, it moved to that plateau to stay, though I always wondered if I were truly there. I could feel myself getting stronger, standing up to the rigours of the day, going to bed at a later hour, resting better. There were so many positives that far outweighed the negatives. And yet all it would take was one regressive day and there would be more questions than answers. With self-talk I was able to rationalize about why I was having a down day. I may or may not have rationalized accurately, but it would satisfy me and keep me from running to see the physician each and every time. I can't begin to guess how many more doctor visits I would have had otherwise.

I had many guides along the way in the form of my medical team, but they were not with me by the hour to help me when I was slipping backwards. Even if they had been, based on my experience their advice would have been that I should set up camp as I needed some rest. If I questioned them about how long I needed to stay in camp and rest, their answer would have been, "Who knows? Maybe days, months, years. Maybe you will never be well enough to complete the climb."

Progression and regression became a way of life until I started to see considerable progression and, indeed, reached a plateau in my health that I identified as the summit.

This analogy of mountain climbing and reaching a summit has taken on new meaning in my life. As I write, I look out at the beautiful, snowcapped Coast Mountains on the horizon. When I look at the highest peak, I associate my ten years of climbing to health with that peak. It was a long, adventurous climb with many obstacles and unknowns along the way.

However, as I look at those peaks I suddenly feel I have climbed not one but a series of mountains, the most significant being my

Commitment to Health program. Frankly, I would choose the highest peak for this accomplishment. It took not only a commitment, but also the strong-mindedness to continue the climb each and every day. Having reached the summit, the Commitment to Health remains an ongoing daily activity to stay on top. Does it not make sense to think that over a lifetime we are climbing mountains all the time, only at different levels?

I am now able to reflect on my lifetime and think of milestone accomplishments, and it reinforces the idea that I have reached many summits and have not just been on one big lifetime climb with an unattainable summit. This image of life as a series of climbs and summits is a positive one, as many of the summits I have reached came in relatively short time frames and these successes made me feel good about myself.

Since I conquered the ten-year climb that followed my accident, there have been other, shorter climbs with their own stresses and constraints. For instance, one September morning in 1995 Sasha asked me what was wrong with my right eye.

"Nothing," I said. "Why?"

She told me that my right eyelid was lower than my left. I checked in a mirror and she was right. But I had just had a shave – why, I wondered, had I not noticed it then? I decided I didn't look too closely at myself in the mirror, but there was a great deal of observation over the next few days. I found that in the latter part of the day, the droop in my eyelid was more pronounced than in the morning. I was concerned about how long this condition had existed, but then I realized that Sasha would have noticed it immediately even if I had not.

I made an appointment to see my physician. Dr. Bull reserved comment on what the condition might be, but he did say that he was going to have me see a neurologist immediately. My first appointment was on October 5, 1995, and after some questions the neurologist, Dr. John MacFadyen, proceeded with an examination of my eyes, yet another new experience for me. Dr. MacFadyen told me that he would be carrying out some tests over the next few weeks to confirm his suspicions, but he told me he was quite certain I had ocular myasthenia gravis. He booked me for an appointment at Chilliwack General Hospital the following week and told me that at this appointment he would give me an injection that would determine if my symptoms were the result of this disorder.

When I arrived at the hospital for the appointment, I was immediately ushered into an examination room with a bed. Dr. MacFadyen and a registered nurse arrived soon after. The doctor asked me to lie down and asked the nurse to observe the eyelid. After the injection, the nurse exclaimed, "My God, I have never seen anything like it. The eyelid is raised." I assumed that this confirmed the doctor's suspicions about my problem.

I later learned that I had undergone what is called a Tensilon test. The doctor injects edrophanium chloride to determine if a patient's symptoms are due to myasthenia gravis or not. Two milligrams are injected intravenously as a test dose. If no definite relief of symptoms has occurred after thirty to forty-five seconds, a further eight milligrams are injected. Witnessing a positive Tensilon test is one of the most dramatic experiences in medicine. Eyelids may spring back into open position. The flip side to this test was that I did not sense or feel anything happen. As well, the eyelid slid back to its droopy position in no time, and again I was not sensitive to this.

On this same visit I had blood tests that were sent to University Hospital at UBC for culture. The results confirmed that I had myasthenia gravis.

The last test, also at Chilliwack General Hospital, was a pulmonary function test, which involved my deep inhaling and exhaling into an apparatus that measured lung capacity. This test was performed to confirm whether any muscles were affected in the lungs. Fortunately this test showed that I was in a healthy range.

I was put on medication and it did not take long for my eyelid to raise to its normal position. I was elated. By the time I saw Dr. Bull again, he was aware of the diagnosis and confirmed that I had a rare, non-communicable disease. He went on to tell me that I should not start seeking other medical help or spend a lot of money treating this condition. He informed me that the late Aristotle Onassis had had myasthenia gravis and he spent a fortune trying to find a cure, with no success. This did not give me any more concern than I already had. I had discovered that myasthenia gravis is a neuromuscular disorder characterized by weakness and abnormal fatigue of the voluntary muscles. The first authenticated account involved a man named Sir Thomas Willis in 1685. Though it is not curable, the disorder does respond to treatment in the form of specific medications, as well as to surgical and other medical procedures. In severe cases, almost all the muscles may be affected by the weakness, including those involved in breathing. In some cases the onset of symptoms may follow stress, emotional upset, infection, surgery, or administration of neuromuscular blocking agents.

After reviewing material I received from the Myasthenia Gravis Association of BC, I have come to grips with the seriousness of the condition. How rare is it? Its occurrence is estimated to be from forty-three to eighty-four people per million of the population. Is it any wonder I originally asked myself, why me? After learning what causes the onset of symptoms, is it any wonder that I asked myself if it was due to the prolonged stress, emotional upset, and the multiple surgeries I underwent over the ten years of my disability? Only those who are specialists in this area may come to some conclusion, but for the present, I as a layperson feel that some or all of the factors that may trigger myasthenia gravis are present in my case and could have been contributing factors.

I have also learned that if a case of ocular myasthenia gravis stays confined to the eye for a period of two years, it generally will not spread from that area. After passing that anniversary in November 1997 I was happy that the condition was still confined to my eye. Earlier in the year I was taken off medication and the droopy eyelid showed up again. This proved that the medication was helping and that the condition was still with me. I am hoping that it will not manifest itself in any other part of my body, but as with everything else, time will tell.

A few months before the drooping eyelid first appeared, on July 12, 1995, I had an appointment with Dr. Clive Duncan, an orthopaedic surgeon in Vancouver. As I mentioned in chapter 18, in 1994 I had a series of X-rays on my hip and consulted with a rheumatologist. I had been having problems with my right leg and hip. Not only was there pain, but I was also having difficulty walking. I was progressively favouring my right side. Now Dr. Duncan did an exhaustive examination and though he told me I was not yet a candidate for a hip replacement, he would see me on a periodic basis to keep an eye on things.

I was able to get around with the help of a cane, but there were times when the pain was severe, especially when a certain type of weight or pressure was exerted on the hip. Nevertheless, the pain was not as constant as what I had previously felt, and I had built up a high pain-tolerance level. I had many pain-management techniques up my sleeve, which helped on difficult days.

Six months later I had deteriorated considerably and Dr. Duncan scheduled me for surgery on May 7, 1996. (I want to digress for a moment here and emphasize that if you are involved in a motor vehicle accident and your condition after the accident is markedly different from that before the accident, there is something wrong. You should seek information on possible long-term effects. If you have an insurance claim, do not settle until you are well. Even then, something of a long-term nature could still show up after a settlement. In my case, damage to the hip that ultimately resulted in a hip replacement was no doubt a result of the 1991 accident. The extent of the damage became clear after I had settled the claim, yet I was suffering pain at the time of the settlement. I discuss this issue in greater detail in Chapter 20.)

In the month prior to surgery I visited the Red Cross and had a blood bank set up so I would have my own blood to use in the event that it was needed during surgery. This was a precautionary move and, I believe, a wise one, as whose blood is better than your own should it be required? As well, I had tried to be a blood donor over the years, but because I had a history of a thyroid condition I had been ruled out. Now I was pleased that at the very least I could act as my own donor.

Prior to surgery I was also put on an iron supplement. By this time, after what I had been through, I felt as if I were built of iron, but I did not question the decision.

I will not describe the hospital and surgical procedures in detail as I have covered these subjects before. However, there were two items that stand out for me. My anxiety level heightened in the days before surgery, as I had been through considerable trauma in the past. Although I had total faith in Dr. Duncan, I could not help worrying about the implications of yet another major reconstruction in a vital part of my body. I was no longer in pain from my neck problem, but now a major invasion was about to take place in another part of my body that was closely related to my aerobic walking program. I was determined that this activity not be curtailed. I could live with it if I were slowed down, but I would find it difficult to give up walking. All I could do was hope that it would turn out well.

The other interesting item took place the evening before surgery. I had been admitted to Vancouver General Hospital on May 6, 1996, because of the distance from our home to the hospital. From my past experience I knew there would be a steady stream of medical personnel visiting me, so at first I saw nothing different when Dr. E. Masterson arrived. He was an orthopaedic surgeon from Dublin, doing his fellowship with Dr. Duncan in reconstructive surgery. We had a brief chat and then he said his visit had a purpose. He told me that Dr. Duncan was participating in a scientific study of a new cement for hip replacements. This new cement had been developed because doctors were having some problems with the old cement and hoped that the new one was a superior product. Dr. Masterson said that I had been chosen as a candidate for this study if I was willing to participate. If I agreed to participate, there was no guarantee that I would end up with the new cement. Both the old and new cements were being used in surgery so that there would be a measure for comparison. Dr. Masterson told me that in the operating room, when it came time to use the cement, the surgeon would open an envelope and only then would he know if he was to use the old or new cement. I would not be told which cement had been used.

I was caught completely off guard and after a short discussion we agreed that he should leave me to think it over for a time. He also left the authorization documents that I would need to sign if I wanted to participate in the study. Here I was, the night before surgery, with a lot on my mind and now my mind was travelling a mile a minute. I had a lot of questions. I could make it simple and say no and I would automatically be left with the old cement. I could say yes and I could still get the old cement. I had been assured that the new cement was superior, but I could not request its use – only take a chance that I would receive it if I took part in the study. Was there a risk factor in using the old cement? Was there nothing I could do but accept the risk? Did I want to be in a lottery, a game of chance, if I agreed to participate? If I agreed to participate in the study, what would be the long-term effects of always wondering which cement had been used?

By the time I put my thoughts together, Dr. Masterson was back to see me. I told him that I would like to participate in the study and I was comfortable with the chance that I would end up with the new cement as it would be at least as good as the old. He agreed.

I went on to say that when I made a decision, I usually did so knowing the rationale on which the decision was made. In this case, I felt that going with the scientific study was not a problem. It would not bother me if I got the old cement instead of the new, as taking the chance would have been my decision. However, not knowing which cement was used would always be a question mark in my mind, a piece of unfinished business.

Dr. Masterson's response was, "You appear to be mature about your thinking and I am satisfied with your response. Should you go ahead with the study, we will tell you whether you got the old or the new cement." I signed the necessary documents, we shook hands, and he wished me the very best and said he would see me the next day.

The morning of surgery had its anxious moments. Having previous surgery does not necessarily prepare you for the next operation, and this is an experience we would be pleased never to have to undergo in our life. It is a serious commitment from yourself and the medical team, but I was fully prepared to put my life in their hands. It was a comfort to have Sasha with me before I was wheeled away to the operating room.

I had a long wait before I entered the operating room, but various staff came by to reassure me that it would not be too much longer. The only thing I recall from the operating room was the sound of surgical tools working on my hip. The cutting sounds were not comforting, but the spinal anaesthetic obviously did its job as I know I tried to move but was motionless.

When Dr. Duncan visited me in my room after surgery, he told me that the operation had been successful. My hip had been in bad shape as there was no cartilage and it had been bone on bone. There was little wonder I had been feeling such pain. The good news was that I had "won the lottery" and received the new cement. It was a great day for me.

I was overjoyed when I was able to stand up on the second day. It was only for moments and I was fully supported by nurses, but it was a good experience. My recovery was slower than expected and I later learned there were discussions about discharging me to a rehabilitation centre before I went home. Both Dr. Duncan and Dr. Masterson, as well as all the hospital staff, were most supportive during my convalescence, and I took a turn for the better and went home on the twelfth day after surgery. The time slipped by quickly. Sasha stayed in town for a few days and then went home until I was discharged. We talked on the phone every day and she did some networking after she got home, calling family, friends, and former business colleagues, many of whom came in to visit me. So many former colleagues came by that I felt as if I were back in business.

The hundred-kilometre trip home was a long one, and then I had to face a series of stairs when I arrived home. Our home is multilevel, and the first set of seven stairs was an experience. The second set of eight was a double experience. The third set of six was a relief, as I could go straight on to bed. My short training session on the use of crutches proved to be helpful.

I tested myself daily with the crutches and it was not too long before I made it to our main gate, 500 feet from our house. With this first trip I knew that my walking program was back on track, albeit on crutches. I was moving ever so slowly, but move I did. I was given a list of exercises to do each day. Some of them were not easy, but I persevered as I wanted to get better. I attended a few physiotherapy sessions and the physiotherapist, who felt I was doing well on my own, gave me the option of carrying on by myself, which I did. I was able to wean myself off the crutches in about three months and by November I discontinued using the cane. I was back on my own two feet. What a feeling!

The scientific study necessitated that I have periodic check-ups as well as X-rays in the first year. All appeared to be well and though I still tended to favour my right leg at times, I was assured that it was only a matter of time till the muscle healed.

Have I reached the summit? Are hip problems and myasthenia gravis behind me? I do not know, but I am happy with the view from the current plateau and hope I can stay here for the future.

Chapter 20

CAREER CARVE-OUT

One of the major stressors I faced during my ten years of dealing with the neck injury was giving up my job. The May 1989 phone call from my employer, when I was told that I would have to relinquish my position if I was not able to return to work within the six-month time frame, was traumatic, to say the least. So were the days that followed as I came to the realization that here I was, in the prime of life, out of a job. Or, rather, I was out of the management position I had held in this company. In the life insurance business I would never be out of a job if I could return to work. For this reason I continued to renew my licence to sell insurance as the years went by. I don't know whether I shall hang up my shingle again. That depends on my ability to function and operate a business. I do not want to put myself in a position where my health would regress because of the demands of business.

The stress resulting from this phone call could have been much worse, but fortunately at the time of my accident I had short- and long-term disability income replacement coverage. This coverage was part of the wages and benefits package in my contract with the company and I took it for granted. I had not imagined I would use the coverage in the way I did and for the length of time I did, but I can uncategorically state that had it not been for this coverage, we would not have been able to maintain the standard of living that we had come to enjoy. Indeed, the policy probably saved me from financial ruin. While I no longer had the ability to increase my income from year to year, this policy insured that I did have an income. I did not have to start diminishing my hard-earned resources or depleting the reserves I had set aside for retirement. Moreover, I could meet my existing financial obligations.

Payments from a long-term disability insurance policy generally stop when you reach age sixty-five. What is significant is that any resources you built up to the time of your disablement will have been protected and left to accumulate until the time the disability income ceases. If you suffer a prolonged disability, you could still face seriously decreased income at retirement depending on the amount of capital and other resources you held in reserve at the time you were injured or became ill.

I could not foresee that my employer's phone call was the start of a long-term disability claim that would continue till I was sixty-five. Who would have thought it would take me ten years, from age fifty-five to sixty-five, to recover from a double rear-ended collision, with all my opportunity to continue to work and to increase my income wiped out?

When I came to the realization there would be no quick fix, I did my utmost to take control of the situation and maintain an interest in what was happening to me. The rude awakening was that suddenly my whole lifestyle was changing and there was absolutely no escape. To this day I have not fully accepted the loss of those years. I doubt that I ever will.

On June 24, 1994, I wrote in my diary: "As I reflect on the last few years and my career interruption, there continues to be an empty feeling for not having had the opportunity to do the many things I had planned for at a very critical period of my life.

"Having been taken away from my work in the fashion that I was is an unforgettable experience, leaving behind incomplete and unfinished goals which I had set out for myself. Silently my career goal was to have the biggest marketing operation in the company. This career objective was very strong within me and I knew I could do it. It is unbelievable how in a split second one's career can be shattered, crumbled, and you have absolutely no control over your destiny."

I want to emphasize that we never anticipate disaster. We take it for granted that nothing will happen to us...until it happens. This is fate in the truest form. It offers no warnings in advance. We do not anticipate disaster, we can't prevent it, and generally speaking, it happens suddenly. The hospitals and private care homes are full of disaster cases and patients requiring various levels of care. As I have been in the life insurance business, I believe I have some expertise in this topic. For me, disaster was a "Career Carve-Out." It could have been "Total Financial Ruin." I could have become paralyzed.

Something could have gone wrong on the operating table and I might not have lived to tell my story.

If we take our life cycle and break it up into decades, it is startling how little time we have to make a mark in our career. An individual only has six and a half decades before he or she is headed for the pension rolls. As well, it is almost certain in North American society that the better part of the first two or two and a half decades are spent in dependency. This is when we do our learning and are moulded, in one way or another, with definitive imprints that shape who and what we are in the years to come.

The next four decades are spent on our own, possibly sharing the load with a spouse or partner. These working decades are demanding as we must provide for all the necessities of life, one of which, shelter, is a major drain on the budget. This is also the time when many people decide to have children and raise a family. These critical years fly by quickly. If you are raising a family, by the time your children have grown up you are already in your last decades in the work force.

Another major area that must be attended to during this period is, ironically, retirement. It is important early in one's working and earning years to learn to start paying yourself a portion of your earnings, setting it aside for retirement. During our working years we work for money. We put it away so it will grow, and when the time comes the role is reversed and the money will work for us. There's nothing magical about this. It just requires the discipline of getting started early in life. If you plan ahead and provide for yourself in this way, you will have the financial freedom to be independent when you retire. Being dependent at that stage of life does not offer too much security and the result is a lifestyle that may be marginal or worse.

For many people there is a complete turnaround during the last decades of life and they are back to a dependency beyond their control. This may be due to sickness, injury, or just the effects of old age. For other people, this turnaround comes sooner. Many people face major disruptions due to illness or prolonged disability during their lifetime. The disruptions can be so traumatic that they totally change one's life and alter a career path. In some cases this may even be a good thing.

The turnaround came sooner than expected for me. I entered the life insurance business as an agent at the age of thirty-one in May 1962.

At the time of my accident I was manager of a life insurance brokerage agency. I was peaking in my career, but in a split second all that I had planned for at this stage of life was disrupted. I was suddenly dealt health problems beyond my control, an infringement on the smooth life cycle. It was a nightmare to find myself struggling with my daily routine, which in the past was "all in a day's work." I was overwhelmed by a problem I could not solve, even though I had been a diligent problem solver in the past. The difference now was that it was a health problem beyond my power to resolve. It did not help that I didn't know the exact nature of the injury and the potentially serious effect it could have on me. I could not understand how it drained my energy and took a heavy toll by day's end.

In my case, I was in the last decade of my career when I had my first surgery. Little did I know then what kind of time was going to be carved out of my working years. And these were working years at the prime of my life. This interruption of my life cycle would totally alter my lifestyle and, ultimately, affect the planning I had done for my retirement years.

This leads me to one important point for anyone who suffers an injury from an accident. A serious aspect of personal injury is the possibility of health deterioration in the future. If you settle an insurance claim right away and further injury-related problems appear later, there may be no recourse for further damages. I can recall meeting a lawyer on my daily walks, getting into conversations with him on different occasions, and learning from him that there are situations where injured people try to settle a case too soon. This is where medical experts and legal counsel become involved. It is imperative that medical specialists examine and assess your injuries and predict your short- and long-term outlook. If you find it hard to communicate with an adjuster or feel an adjuster is not looking out for your best interests, seek legal help. Your lawyer will deal with the adjuster and shield you from what can be an intimidating experience. And my main recommendation for anyone involved in an accident is to keep a diary of your problems if you are able. It may be helpful for your doctors or your insurance claim.

Either through ignorance or the fact that I generally handled all my own affairs, I did not immediately seek legal advice after my accident.

As my case was accident related, my doctor kept the provincial insurance corporation informed of my medical situation. My surgeon also provided both short- and long-term observations (I was not aware of these at the time). The insurance adjuster, armed with this information and reports of medical examinations by the insurance corporation's own doctors, used every means possible to persuade me there was nothing wrong with me. The adjuster came up with a settlement offer based on a similar case and sent me a cheque in settlement, as well as the discharge papers to sign.

I was continually getting calls from the adjuster. He pressured me to cash the cheque, as I had not cashed it when I received it. The adjuster insisted that we had to close the case. It could not go on forever. I replied that all I wanted was my health. As soon as I had it I would satisfy him by settling the case. Every month I would get another call from the adjuster. He was not concerned about my health; he simply wanted me to endorse the cheque as he needed to secure his files.

I did not like his tactics and in November 1986 I saw a lawyer, days before the statute of limitations would have run out. From that time on I did not speak with the adjuster again, though I later learned that he had his knuckles rapped due to his aggressive tactics with claimants.

Getting back to the discussion of the life cycle, my accident occurred in what I refer to as the prime time of my working years. What happens to individuals who suffer a major setback during their teen years? Depending on the number of years lost to convalescence, they may well have to redirect their life and may never reach the economic peak they might have achieved had they enjoyed a healthy life.

What about individuals who have just graduated from university, college, or technical school and are either getting into the work force or are already semi-established? A carve-out of even a few years due to disability will have a profound financial impact for the rest of their lives.

Injury or illness could happen in mid-career, at a time when an individual is progressing favourably with great expectations. It does not matter when the interruption occurs during the life cycle; if it happens during the pre-retirement years it will cause unpredictable losses to one's career, lifestyle, and economic wellbeing.

This is not to say that, after recovery, people will not carry on from where they left off or make a successful career change. What I am saying is that, for better or for worse, such a disruption will have a serious impact on an individual. It may well be positive, but in the meantime they may have suffered economic losses to the point that they are in financial ruin.

What I want to stress is that we have no control over our destiny in terms of health. In the insurance business, disability is often referred to as a living death because we can never be certain how long the disability will last or how much money it will require. If it lasts longer than one's resources, it is certain to bankrupt you. I have read many stories of situations where, due to disability, homes were lost because of the owner's inability to maintain the mortgage.

Fortunately there are mechanisms available to provide protection against economic loss due to illness or injury. In my case, I was fortunate to have in place insurance coverage for short- and long-term disability, as I described above.

It is crucial to have as much income replacement insurance as you can afford to protect yourself from financial ruin in the event of disability. Then there is the other aspect – if you make it to what would have been your retirement age on insurance, what do you live on after retirement age?

Having said that, forget about disability for the moment and just think in terms of retirement plans. This is a disaster area for many people who are too busy to plan for the day when they have all that time on their hands and nothing to do. We all know people who were winners in the pre-retirement period but who entered a lost world after they stopped working.

As a result of my disability I have suffered severe financial losses. However, there was a trade-off. The trade-off was that I learned to live and cope with an unknown medical condition over a prolonged period of time and I developed an enriching life of self-knowledge and meaningful projects. I grew personally with the assistance of medical help, reaching plateaus I would never have dreamed of reaching before the accident.

We cannot see the future, but with the power of planning, with insurance policies, retirement savings, and a good To Do List, we can try to prepare for it.

Chapter 21

CAREGIVER

This book could not have been completed without the presence of my caring wife Sasha.

In the split second when I had my accident, her life changed. She went from being a homemaker, a mother, a grandmother to the unfamiliar role of caregiver. One could easily say that a mother's role is that of a caregiver and they would be absolutely correct. However, by going through my disability experience with me, Sasha became a caregiver of a special kind. There is no question in my mind – after living my experience and observing a number of other situations – that caregiving is a specialized field involving vast numbers of family members as well as members of the medical profession.

When we took our marriage vows in October 1953, we did not realize how significant those vows were. When you are first married, you never imagine your married life as anything other than blessed. And blessed we were, with a wonderful family and the adventure of raising our two daughters and four sons. Sasha did a great job of raising six children, and just when in the normal course of things she would have been able to enjoy her grandchildren, in a split second her life and our relationship changed dramatically. She was not a victim, but a victim of circumstance.

In the early stages it was quite apparent that there was something drastically wrong with me. I was not responding to treatment given to whiplash victims and soon I was referred to an orthopaedic surgeon. Even though I tried not to show how troubled I was, it was impossible to hide. I was on a path through the unknown and this in itself created a heavy burden for Sasha. It is one thing to know what you are up against; it is another when you are the caregiver in a situation where you and your charge are helpless. As various members of the family visited, they all tried to be helpful, but how does one help when the medical profession itself is in an uncertain state?

247

More than ever, Sasha was becoming involved in my medical visits, X-rays, blood tests, and physiotherapy sessions. Suddenly she was finding that along with the beginning of my career carve-out, she was seeing a carve-out from her daily routine. I was becoming reliant on her because I was less able to manage on my own, particularly when it came to driving a motor vehicle.

Being the chauffeur for a person in my condition was a nightmare for Sasha. She is the best of drivers, but my neck injury meant that I was more delicate than an eggshell, and no matter how I attempted to brace myself against the motion of the vehicle, it was impossible. An unexpected brake would literally put me through the roof. I would scream from the compounded pain radiating up the back of the neck into the skull. It would have been hard enough to tolerate my condition for a few days, weeks, or even months, but she lived with it for years, and although she operated the vehicle with the greatest care, it was an impossible predicament to be in. Is this what caregiving is all about? Subjecting me, under her eyes, to compounded pain while she has absolutely no control over the situation?

The stresses piled up on me and I found myself on a treadmill of visiting professional people with her at my side. At first I didn't see how involved she was, but I came to realize that she was both living with my problem and hearing a lot of uncertainty from the medical profession. She would take part in discussions with my medical team, only to find that she had made no headway at the end of a visit. Our hopes would rise when a medical person said, "I wish we could do more for you," but then nothing would come of it. Sasha was clearly finding it as difficult to cope with the negatives and uncertainties as I was.

It was hard for me to comprehend the feelings of my caregiver as she sat beside me, listening to the orthopaedic surgeon's recommendation for further treatment. He told us that surgical intervention was required at three levels of the spine and then went on to warn that the possible downside from such surgery was that I could end up in a wheelchair as a quadri- or paraplegic. It was difficult enough for me to hear this when I thought of how young we both were to face such a possibility. When I looked at Sasha, she had literally turned white. I had never seen her this way and I was alarmed.

The surgeon recognized our dilemma and told us to think about it, scheduling a follow-up appointment. But what was there for me to think about? I was in such pain that I would try anything for relief – even the risk of being paralyzed. I knew I was a risk taker, especially if I thought there was an upside chance in my favour.

However, what about the caregiver? Sasha became withdrawn at the thought of my surgery. Her thoughts turned to the possibility that I would become a cripple and she wondered, "How would I manage? We would need a wheelchair and wheelchair access to our home. We would need another vehicle." She thought about how difficult it was for her already. How could she possibly handle such an added burden? If she could not handle the burden, what would she do? Get help in the home? Or leave me in some facility away from home? She had already seen her life greatly altered and she did not see herself as strong enough to deal with me if, heaven forbid, things did not go right.

As these thoughts churned in her mind, she continued to be a caregiver. It is hard to imagine the stress she endured, all the while doing everything possible to hold her composure. How helpless she must have felt when, on a visit to my personal physician, I got out of the car and sat down on the curb, eventually getting up but with no recollection of the incident.

Sasha's job as a caregiver followed me wherever I went. The periods when I was in hospital and out of the house did not lighten her load whatsoever. There was the anxiety and burden of booking me into the hospital, the worry of surgery, and then the time away from home to visit me daily while I was in the hospital – all of it done with a smile.

I underwent every procedure with high hopes that it was a step on the road to recovery. However, I only had to look at my caregiver to see how much she was suffering and how helpless she felt. There is no question of the trauma I went through during surgery. However, I cannot imagine how it must have been for Sasha on the day of surgeries, waiting anxiously for that phone to ring to tell her of a successful surgery. Then she would come to the hospital and be at my bedside when I opened my eyes. The worry she went through as she watched me all wired up and monitored was a frightful experience, and then she had to worry about whether everything would stay stable and proper healing would take place.

Although my daily needs were not excessive, the demands on Sasha's time did not diminish and she had the added burden of maintaining a household and looking after a calendar of events on my behalf. Even as I moved slowly from plateau to plateau, Sasha's role did not change. It was a routine that was there day in and day out. The stress of everyday living drained me, but I was figuratively in a cocoon, doing what I could to exist, self-managing myself as well as taking part in any activities within my limitations. All of the other responsibilities fell on my caregiver. It was these demands on her on a continued, sustained basis that created a pressure cooker.

How long can a person be expected to carry such additional stress? There is no answer and therein was the difficulty. There was no way of knowing how long this would continue. When I discussed my various stages of health, I often referred to how different it was not seeing a glimmer of light at the other end of the tunnel. Sasha was also not seeing any light. If there were a glimmer of light on occasion, relief would come with it. As I suffered rollercoaster pain, Sasha had some severe rollercoaster emotions and down times. She could see herself getting old caregiving or being unable to cope. She suffered a tremendous loss of enjoyment of life and yet we had everything our hearts desired except for my health. As Sasha would say, it was not easy living from day to day observing someone in such pain.

We did not expect that my disability would take such a heavy toll on Sasha. Her emotions were running high and slowly anger crept in. Is it any wonder? Here we were after more than thirty years of marriage - something must have held us together that long, but because of my health problem and her involved role as caregiver, our marital relationship was becoming strained. Although I may have thought there were no cracks showing on my part, I was becoming short tempered – out of character but understandable under the circumstances – and occasionally my temper would get out of control and I would unnecessarily inflict deep wounds on my caregiver. The same thing was happening to Sasha, and we unwittingly developed some retaliatory situations that only added to the stress we were already enduring. This came about slowly and subtly and was with us before we knew it. At first it was difficult to understand how we had allowed this to happen, but on reflection, there was nothing we could have done differently. It

JERRY OLYNYK

was a matter of two people being held prisoners, hostage within their own bodies, and doing their best to live within the confines of the space to which they were limited. We worked to avoid confrontations and I would feel guilty when they happened as I knew not only that my caregiver cared, but that it was not in her nature to have such confrontations.

I have no doubt that our commitment to communication helped us tremendously during some difficult days. Communication may address and resolve some problems, but the problems from within the caregiver are of a different kind and only those who have been in similar circumstances can fully understand them.

Is this what the marriage vows are all about? I think not, but fate can play some tricks and Sasha was smack in the middle of a traumatic experience of her own. Her anxiety levels were kept high just doing her best to try and look after me. What a burden to put on a person, and though she was the healthy one, she was quickly losing her own health from worry.

As I was seeing my personal physician and specialists on a continuing basis, Sasha was sharing her heavy burden with her personal physician. When it reached the point where the physician felt she was no longer helping, she recommended that Sasha see a psychologist. We discussed it, I encouraged her to do so, and she made an appointment. It turned out to be not only a timely visit, but most helpful as well. Sasha told me she was given the opportunity to relate her story, her concerns, her anxiety, her worries, and her problems of coping on a daily basis with my condition.

The psychologist was to be commended for her quick comprehension of Sasha's problems and her response to them. When she explained that all of her problems and concerns were normal under the circumstances, Sasha felt tremendous relief. It was obvious that along with the heavy load she was coping with, she had also developed a guilt feeling about what she perceived as her inadequacy in helping me.

It took only one visit to put her on the right track to being a caregiver with much less pressure on her. The psychologist suggested that she would like to meet with both of us on a return visit, but Sasha did not feel the need for a follow-up interview.

251

Over time I recognized that Sasha needed some time of her own. I did not begrudge her this time. In fact, I encouraged her to take it, but she could not escape a feeling of guilt as she wondered how I would manage on my own. We arranged for Sasha to get away periodically for a few days at a seaside resort or a visit with family. During these breaks I would stay at home and Sasha would call daily. Fortunately we got by without any emergencies, and she had a chance to rejuvenate herself.

I made sure that the two of us got out together for dinners, the occasional movie, a live play, a symphony concert, and strolls along the seawall by the ocean. If the person in care is in any way able to take part in some activities away from home, it provides a critical balance for the caregiver. By the same token, getting out, even on a limited basis, is also therapeutic for the person in care. There were many times when I suggested we go out, even though I was suffering excruciating pain all the while.

I did everything possible to make her load easier, but she bottled up her burden and her worries within herself, sharing them with no one as she felt obligated to see me through. In many ways her worries and concerns were no different from mine, however, when you are a caregiver, they take on a different significance. How could she discuss her concerns with me when she saw that I was barely getting through each day? How could she reveal what she was feeling when she saw I already had more than enough to deal with?

She felt helpless about her ability to help me. I often felt the same way as I was so reliant on her. Not for a moment did I feel she was inadequate, but I did not know how to make her believe that. As her caregiving stretched into years with what seemed to be no progress, she felt more and more doubt about whether anything she was doing for me helped. It was not the stress of the caregiving that was troubling near as much as the stress and worry of my health condition. I gave to her in every way possible, but was hampered by my limitations. And my giving was altogether different from what Sasha gave to me as a caregiver. My dependence on her was so great that she had to reprogram all her household duties to revolve around my priority needs, demands far above and beyond the call of duty.

One may ask when a role is beyond the call of duty in a marriage. In normal, healthy, marital relationships one may expect some ups and

252

downs, however, a caregiver role such as Sasha had was far beyond the call of duty, in my opinion. And I do not believe she acted out of a call to duty. She was motivated by the loving, caring relationship she had with me. I had always been a primary focus in her life (as she had been in mine), but there is a big difference between caring and caregiving. Sasha accepted my needs and rose to the occasion without complaint. Somehow, with the extra load she was carrying, she would continue to give that caring smile. At times the caring smile was noticeably strained. This was usually when she was emotionally drained. She was having her nerves tested to the outer limits.

We had our outings, our social life, and she had her day or few days to escape, but afterwards she always returned to the same set of circumstances. And prolonged stress with no hope in sight, compounded by negative self-talk, is naturally going to take its toll. I did my best to understand what she was coping with. However, it is impossible to get inside another person. Conversely, as a caregiver she only had to look at me to know how I was feeling.

We were receiving sympathy from all sides, from friends and family, and all of it was gratefully acknowledged, but in my opinion it was Sasha, the caregiver, who could have used this support and positive reinforcement because she had the ability to respond. With me it was like water off a duck's back. Whatever stage I was at was my condition at the time and I just had to cope with it – no amount of sympathy would change it. But Sasha was also suffering and sympathy and encouragement could help her.

We had one appointment with a family counsellor in 1994. Both Sasha and I were able to tell our story, what we were doing, how we were coping. We got everything out in the open. After a lengthy interview the counsellor complimented us on how we were dealing with the matter at hand. She could not offer any further suggestions, wished us luck, gave us each a hug, and we were on our way.

It was gratifying that a professional person recognized we had matters under control, but it was disappointing for Sasha as the counsellor could not offer her any further advice on her role as a caregiver. Sasha was searching for something more than what she got, and the failure to find it had a negative effect on her thinking. She wondered why she had agreed to see the counsellor and waste our time,

253

especially as she had doubted that there was any new help to be had. I, on the other hand, was always willing to give these medical appointments a try in the hope that somewhere, somehow we would find a way to help my caregiver make her job a little easier. I also felt that although there may not have been tangible help, indirectly the session was valuable because of the positive assessment and encouragement from the counsellor.

The reality was that we had matters under control as best we could, we were coping as best we could. Under the circumstances, both of us had adjusted to a lifestyle that revolved around my physical capabilities. Our marriage had been sound and now, because of my disability, had been tested, which in its own way strengthened the marital bond. We had a home environment that left nothing to be desired. We had everything except my health, which in turn affected the health of my caregiver.

After such a lengthy fight, my strongest hope was that she would be able to hold herself together. It was not easy on me when she told me how my prolonged illness was dragging her down. I did everything I could to be supportive, but I had my limitations. I even went so far as to assure her that to save her health I could not stand in her way if she decided to go her way and live in peace away from a struggling being.

However, after thirty-plus years of marriage there was a hidden force working silently on both of us. The marriage vows are strong and although I will never know how strong an influence they were, I believe the words "Till death do us part" were a silent saviour. We exhausted all our resources and learned to live and cope with the most difficult health uncertainties. More than thirty years of love and devotion made it possible for both of us to rise to every occasion. I believe Sasha's caregiving came from being my wife, and all of the emotions that played heavily on her were overruled by one word: LOVE.

With time, as I started to get better, there were noticeable positive changes in terms of stress release. It was a great relief for both of us. Seven years after the accident, Sasha enrolled in a ten-week art course put on by a local artist. It was a positive step in her own recovery process, as she was again able to do one of the things she loved as well as meet new people with a similar interest.

A caregiver is an individual who cares for someone out of LOVE. I received her care out of LOVE. Together we have shared an experience beyond comprehension – an experience of the POWER OF LOVE.

Chapter 22

A LONG JOURNEY
by Sasha Olynyk

Life is full of surprises, good and bad. Little do we realize how events can change our lives around and bring out resources we didn't know we had, testing them in great depth.

The day Jerry called from work to say he had been involved in a traffic accident on the way to work, I did not begin to fathom what lay in store for us both.

The initial fear and concern about the seriousness of the accident gave way to weeks and months of attempting to cope with the lasting effects of this immense, debilitating reality. My husband was a man of great energy and well-being who found his work stimulating and rewarding, but gradually, as the pain level increased despite the medication, the debilitation worsened. To see Jerry trying to cope with his job, his home life, and the lessening resources of his body was difficult to deal with, as I was unable to ease the burden that had been placed upon him by this untimely and unwanted event. How great the gift of good health is to all of us.

As the months slipped by we went through the motions of finding out what could be done, and on a fateful Sunday in 1988 I took Jerry to Lions Gate Hospital emergency. Jerry was now in excruciating pain and could no longer tolerate the daily pain emanating from his neck area. All the rest and medication, the consultations with surgeon and family doctor had reached a point of no return. I felt we had reached an abyss – we couldn't go back but there was nothing ahead of us. Surgery was the only hope, for the second time.

When I originally heard the words "quadri- or paraplegic" as a possible result of surgery, I was stunned and frightened. How in the world would I cope with this frightening possibility by myself? Our home was not built for such a situation and I was not sure I would be able to physically and mentally cope for the rest of our lives with such a demand. I knew that over the long haul I could not do it, and as much as I love my husband, I had to be open with him. It was foolish and useless to do otherwise. We all have within us the strength to do some things, but to do them for a long period would only weaken us both more than we were already.

My emotional level was stressed to the point of requiring psychological help, and physically I was tired beyond reason. It is important to emphasize here that all caregivers must seek medical help early. When the body and mind begin to break down, take heed of the warnings and seek help. Two ill people in such a situation are of no use to anyone. There is help available. My children were supportive, but because they lived away from our home and had their work and families, they could not come in and take over the caregiving duties. I took the opportunities of going away for a day or two to recharge my batteries. More often than not the short time away was helpful, though all it gave me was a little more strength to carry on and cope.

After a visit with a psychologist, which was long overdue, my feelings were of such relief. I cannot explain how this helped me. It allowed me to take myself totally away from the situation in every sense, closing my mind to all thoughts of illness and what was happening to us. This was therapeutic for me and although the time with the psychologist was short, it made a great deal of difference to be able to distance myself from the daily demands that had fallen on my shoulders. The need to cry and cleanse myself of this pain was something that I found I needed. My family, friends, and my doctor were of great support and I can't thank them enough for helping me throughout this lengthy period of my life.

My husband went through so many difficult times before surgery, during recovery, and after. The days and months slipped by, some better than others, and we were always hopeful. There were times of great stress when medications were causing side effects that were frightening. You put great faith in your medical helpers, relying on them to use their knowledge of drugs and guidance to have the body heal. It is always good for the caregiver to request detailed information on prescribed drugs from the pharmacist so you may be alert to any signs that they are not working as they should.

It was to become a long journey, one of learning and coping. I found myself trying to be all things to my husband and I learned that he wanted to do so much more for himself than I thought he was able to do. This was such a great sign that the spirit was willing even though the flesh was weak. It renewed my belief in his full recovery, even though the day he told me that his company could no longer keep his job open for him indefinitely brought more of the many adjustments we were faced with. The medical profession could not guarantee his return to work and our lives took another turn.

A small advertisement in the local newspaper turned my life into something different. The ad was for a home in the country that sounded appealing enough that we decided simply to go for a drive and have a look. Jerry had just been given clearance to take longer trips in the car after having been confined close to home for many months after the second surgery.

We made this trip to the country where high up in the mountains, surrounded by forest, my husband and I felt the peace and healing of our future. We have now come full circle in the sense of starting a new life here in our mountain retreat.

My life here is with nature. The tranquility and cleanliness of the mountain air have restored me more than I can tell you.

I wish any caregiver to have been blessed with this renewal. All situations are different, but keep looking ahead for any glimmer of light at the end of the dark tunnel. Remind yourself constantly why you are where you are, and keep your inner strength constantly renewed in every way you can. It is not easy and you may feel down many times along the way. Get up and keep going for whatever reason you can muster.

Chapter 23

COMMITMENT TO HEALTH

A commitment to a project requires first thought and then the action to keep it in motion until it is finished.

As I reflect on the past fifteen years I see that my lifestyle underwent a complete turnaround. In order to survive I had to make a commitment within myself that I would do everything in my power to fight the battle of the unknown. This battle sapped my energy on a daily basis for years.

During the process of surviving, I made commitments to myself that I would do everything within my power not to feel sorry for myself, to avoid developing the "why me?" syndrome. At various stages I made commitments to keep active within my limitations and to work at projects, even for months on end, to see them through.

Although I did not personally carry out some of the major projects, such as antique vehicle restoration, I felt an incredible sense of accomplishment overseeing the work being done. It is hard to describe how it feels to take on a project such as this, committing yourself to do it and seeing it completed. It would have been easy on so many occasions to pack it in, but what were my alternatives? These commitments were helping me get through some difficult times, and when I thought of giving up I would justify them by asking myself how I could better spend my time. I often thought that these commitments would be a job and a half for a healthy individual, let alone someone in my condition. As it turned out, each and every project I made a commitment to was both successful and highly rewarding.

Prior to my motor vehicle accidents, I made a Commitment to Health and set out on a journey with unknown destination and time frame. The major components of the Commitment to Health were a disciplined walking program along with a change in diet to healthier eating habits. This Commitment to Health program was both initiated and monitored by me, and it has proven to be successful. For one thing, I know it has saved my life. I am sure that surgery would not have been performed had I been as overweight as I was. However, when I started this program it did not have the importance it has for me today. Of all the projects I committed to and completed during these difficult years, my walking program was never in a state of completion. Since I started I have walked over 20,000 miles and, God willing, I have another 20,000 to go. As long as I am able to walk, it is with me for life. The Commitment to Health program turned out to be a "Commitment to Lifelong Health."

Why is it that we find it so difficult to take a few minutes a day in the interest of our personal health? I believe I have proven beyond a doubt that anyone could do the same. Once you become committed, you will never look back and you will provide your body daily with the healthy nourishment and exercise it craves. As I understand it, one drawback to most weight reduction programs is that what is taken off ends up going back on. I found that the simplest, though perhaps the hardest, way to do it is to do it on your own.

In January 1998 the Canadian Fitness and Lifestyle Research Institute reported that two thirds of Canadians do not have a proper exercise program. Another statistic released around the same time was that 51 percent of Canadians are overweight. I challenge all Canadians and people of other countries to make a Commitment to Health and take on the non-prescription drug of aerobic walking. It's a powerful preventative medicine and healer.

Additionally, I urge all readers to treat any important activity in their lives as a total commitment. Make sure the idea that nothing will stop you from continuing and completing a project is firmly implanted in your mind. You may go off track for a while, but the force from within will bring you back. This is the power of commitment.

Glossary

acceleration-deceleration injury. Also known as whiplash, this type of injury to the cervical spine occurs when a person's head is thrown first forwards and then backwards (or vice versa), as in a head-on or rear-ender car accident.

acute pain. Sharp, severe discomfort or agony caused by the stimulation of nerve endings.

acute symptoms. Severe indications of a disease or disorder.

aerobic walking. An exercise program that involves regular exercise such as walking at a rate that increases respiration and heart rate.

anaesthetic. A drug used to eliminate pain. Some form of anaesthetic is used to numb a portion of the body or to put a patient to sleep prior to surgery.

anaesthetist. A medical person trained in the use of anaesthetics.

antibiotics. Drugs used to kill microorganisms or bacteria.

anti-depressant. A drug used to relieve feelings of dejection or discouragement.

anti-inflammatory. A drug that reduces pain and swelling caused by inflammation.

anti-seizure medication. A drug that will prevent a sudden attack or recurrence of pain or disease.

asymptomatic. A condition that presents no indications of disease or injury.

atrophy. A decrease in size or strength or the wasting away of a body part.

biofeedback. A technique in which involuntary body functions (for example, brain waves or blood pressure) are made visible so that a person can exercise control over them.

blood pressure. A measure of the pressure exerted by the body's blood on the walls of the arteries.

bone spur. A projection or outgrowth from a bone.

carotid artery. The principal blood vessel of the neck, which carries blood to the head.

cartilage. An elastic, fibre-containing, connective tissue that is mostly found in joints and respiratory passages.

CAT (computerized transverse tomography) scan. A type of X-ray that shows details of the soft tissue and bones.

cervical collar (soft). A brace that supports the cervical spine or neck. See also Philadelphia collar.

cervical spine. The seven-vertebrae section of the spine in the area of the neck.

cervical spondylosis. Disintegration of a vertebra or vertebrae in the cervical spine.

chiropractic manipulation. A therapy that involves movement and adjustment of the body, particularly the spinal column, to improve the working of the nervous system.

cholesterol. A steroid alcohol present in cells and body fluids to regulate membrane fluidity and metabolism. Too much of the wrong kind of cholesterol can cause hardening of the arteries.

chronic pain. Discomfort or distress that is constant or that recurs frequently and/or lasts for a long time.

compounded pain. Distress that arises from more than one cause.

contusion. A bruise or an injury that does not break the skin.

cortisone. An anti-inflammatory that can be injected into the affected part of the body to relieve pain.

disc. One of the circular structures, consisting of a soft jelly-like substance surrounded by a tough outer skin, that separate vertebrae in the spine.

disc degeneration. A condition in which one or more of the discs in the spine are deteriorating.

diuretic. A drug that increases urination.

elective surgery. A medical procedure or operation that will help a patient but is not urgent.

facet joint. The bone that joins two adjacent vertebrae.

Fiorinal. A pain-killing drug.

herniated disc. A disc that has ruptured, causing the internal contents to squeeze out and possibly press on a nerve root.

hyperextension/hyperflexion injuries. Injuries that occur when the spine is bent backwards (extension) and then forwards (flexion), as during a car accident.

hypertension. Persistently and abnormally high blood pressure.

Inderal. A drug often used to combat hypertension.

Indocid. An anti-inflammatory drug.

inflammation. Pain, swelling, and increased temperature caused by an injury as the body works to eliminate foreign bodies or damaged tissue.

internist. A physician who specializes in the diagnosis and medical (non-surgical) treatment of diseases of adults.

intravenous. Within a vein, or a procedure occurring within a vein. For example, an intravenous injection is an injection into a vein.

invasive procedure. A medical procedure that involves entering the body, whether through an incision or through an instrument being inserted into the spine or a vein.

isometric exercises. Exercises in which muscles are contracted in resistance to a pressure.

isotonic exercises. Exercises in which muscles are contracted with movement but without resisting pressure.

Lasix. A diuretic drug.

ligament. The fibrous tissue that connects bones or cartilages and supports joints.

magnetic resonance imaging. A noninvasive test that produces computerized images of internal body tissues and allows doctors to diagnose problems.

manipulative treatment. A physical therapy in which joints are moved beyond their comfortable limit of motion.

meditation. A pain-management technique in which the patient focuses his or her mind on positive thoughts or on anything other than the pain.

metabolism. The physical and chemical processes by which, for example, food is transformed into energy for use by a human body. Also, the total processes that keep the body functioning.

myelogram. A medical procedure in which dye is injected into the spine.

nerve. A fibrous cord that conveys impulses between a part of the body and the central nervous system

neurological. Having to do with the nerves or the nervous system.

neurologist. A physician specializing in the diagnosis and treatment of neurological problems.

neuromuscular. Relating to nerves and muscles.

neuroradiologist. A medical specialist who uses radiant energy (i.e., X rays or radiation) in the treatment of diseases of the nervous system.

neurosurgeon. A doctor who specializes in operations on the nervous system - nerves, the brain, or the spinal cord.

non-communicable. A disease that cannot be passed from one person to another.

ocular myasthenia gravis. A disease of the eye with symptoms that include progressive weakness of the muscles with no signs of atrophy and no noticeable pain.

organic pain. Pain arising from an organ or organs.

orthopaedic surgeon. A surgeon specializing in the correction or prevention of problems in the skeletal system.

osteoarthritis. Degeneration of bones and cartilage at the joints, accompanied by pain or stiffness.

outpatient. A patient who comes to a hospital or clinic for treatment or tests but does not occupy a bed or stay overnight.

paralysis. The inability to control muscles voluntarily due to nerve or muscle damage.

pharmacology. The science that studies the properties and reactions of drugs and their action on living systems, especially with relation to their medical use.

Philadelphia collar. A hard brace that supports the head and neck without allowing any movement.

physician. A medical practitioner or doctor.

physiology. The study of living organisms, their parts, and the chemical and physical functions and processes involved.

physiotherapy. Physical therapy or the treatment of disease by physical and mechanical means like massage, exercise, water, light, heat, and electricity.

pre-existing condition. A medical problem that existed before a disease or injury.

prognosis. A forecast regarding the time limit for or extent of recovery from an injury or illness.

psychiatrist. A physician who specializes in the study, treatment, and prevention of mental illness.

psychologist. A specialist who studies the mind and mental processes.

pulmonary function. The action of the lungs.

radiologist. A physician specializing in the treatment and diagnosis of disease by using radiant energy (i.e., X rays or radiation).

regressive treatment. Medical care that causes a return of symptoms or a return to an earlier state.

rehabilitation. Restoring an ill or injured person to health or restoring a diseased or injured organ or other body part to healthy function.

residual symptoms. Symptoms that remain after an injury is healed or a disease is cured.

rheumatologist. A doctor specializing in rheumatic conditions, which are any of a variety of disorders involving inflammation and degeneration of connective tissues like joints, muscles, tendons, etc.

scar tissue. The connective tissue that forms a scar, the mark remaining after a wound has healed.

sedative. A drug that calms or tranquilizes the user.

self-hypnosis. A form of pain management that involves putting one's self in a passive, sleeplike state.

self talk. Our internal dialogue, the messages we give ourselves, which can be positive or negative.

soft tissue. The collective name for body tissues including muscular, connective, and fibrous tissues as opposed to bones.

spinal fusion. A medical procedure in which a piece of bone is inserted between two vertebrae.

surgeon. A doctor who specializes in treating disease and injury through operations.

symptomatic condition. A disease that can be identified by specific, perceptible symptoms.

TENS device. A pain-management device that uses electrical impulses to relieve pain by stimulating the body to produce natural painkillers and by overriding the symptoms of pain.

Tensilon test. A test for myasthenia gravis in which a solution of Tensilon (edrophonium chloride) is injected and the eye muscles' weakness should decrease.

traction. A pulling force exerted on the skeleton or a skeletal structure, like the spine or a bone.

trapezius muscle. One of the two large, flat, triangular muscles on either side of the upper back.

trauma. A wound or injury, whether physical or mental/emotional.

vertebrae. The thirty-three bones of the spinal column.

visualization. A pain-management technique that involves creating positive mental images.

voluntary muscle. One of the muscles that can be moved at will. For example, the muscles that open and close the hand.

whiplash. See acceleration/deceleration injuries.